Nursing:
The Career of a Lifetime

Shirley H. Fondiller, EdD, RN, FAAN
and
Barbara J. Nerone, APR

NLN Press • New York
Pub. No. 14-2695

Copyright © 1995
National League for Nursing Press
350 Hudson Street, New York, NY 10014

The views expressed in this publication represent the views of the authors and do not necessarily reflect the official views of the National League for Nursing.

Library of Congress Cataloging-in-Publication Data

Fondiller, Shirley H.
    Nursing : the career of a lifetime / Shirley H. Fondiller and
Barbara J. Nerone.
        p.   cm.
    Pub. no. 14-2695.
    Includes bibliographical references and index.
    ISBN 0-88737-655-X
    1. Nursing—Vocational guidance—United States.   I. Nerone,
Barbara J.   II. Title.
RT82.F55   1995
610.73′06′9—dc20   95-24792
                                                                              CIP

This book was set in Galliard and Garamond by Publications Development Company, Crockett, Texas. The editor and designer was Nancy Jeffries. Northeastern Press, Waymart, Pennsylvania, was the printer and binder. The cover was designed by Lauren Stevens. Photo on page 115, by Cathy Chang, courtesy of National League for Nursing.

Printed in the United States of America

"We must be learning all our lives . . . every year we know more of the great secrets of Nursing. It is a noble calling but *we* must *make* it so."

Florence Nightingale
In a letter of December 23, 1896
to the nurses at the Waltham
   Training School

About the Authors

Shirley H. Fondiller, EdD, RN, FAAN, an internationally known journalist, educator, and historian, is cofounder and principal of Publishing for Health Dimensions (*phd*), an editorial service for nurses and health professionals. She is an adjunct associate professor at Teachers College, Columbia University. In addition to her longtime interest in career counseling, she has published extensively in the health field. Dr. Fondiller has written monographs for leading private foundations, historiographies of nursing organizations, and scripts for the broadcast media.

Barbara J. Nerone, APR, has a broad background in the communications field. She has written and edited articles for nursing journals as well as publications of national associations and service agencies. For two decades, she served as executive editor of *Imprint,* the journal of the National Student Nurses' Association. Elected to the Counselors Academy of the Public Relations Society of America, she is cofounder and principal of Publishing for Health Dimensions (*phd*).

Contents

Contents

Contents

Preface

Over one hundred years ago, modern nursing entered American life. Although the profession's pioneers of that period were remarkable women, it is doubtful that they could have envisioned the circuitous and sometimes difficult journey that nurses would travel in achieving their mission and earning the recognition of society. Nursing, however, has survived over the decades, and has grown in stature and popularity as an exciting career choice for many young women and men.

The marked transformation of nursing in the nineties would be a bit overwhelming to the profession's early leaders. But probably no more than how we today may reflect on potential changes in the approaching 21st century.

Science fiction stimulates our imagination about things to come as do all those "far out" predictions which surprisingly might be right on target. Yet, who in their wildest dreams can truly envision what the high tech revolution will bring, particularly in the area of health care.

This book has been designed to give you a comprehensive picture of contemporary nursing—its expectations and recent trends. It also will give you a glimpse into the future and the new look anticipated in nursing roles. We hope that it will answer many of your questions, and encourage you to join the profession.

Acknowledgments

This book represents a living history of the contributions of many of today's nurses who willingly shared their experiences in professional nursing. We are grateful for their stories, which graphically show the satisfaction they derive in their work and the diverse settings—clinical, academic, and other areas—where nurses practice.

A special thank you goes to the *American Journal of Nursing* for granting permission to reproduce some of the vignettes which first appeared in the "Job Focus" feature by Shirley Fondiller in 1991, and have since been updated.

We also appreciate the valuable resource material available from university and private libraries, as well as data on educational programs supplied by the National League for Nursing.

Our gratitude is extended to the numerous national and international organizations and agencies that provided up-to-date information on their programs and opportunities for nurses.

Finally, we wish to acknowledge Nancy Jeffries for her editorial skill and infinite patience in helping to prepare the work in its present form.

Introduction

There must be something intriguing about becoming a professional nurse. People like to read about nurses, see them in action in films or numerous television soap operas, and follow them for long periods in a popular television series like the addictive *Mash*. Whether depicted as fact or fiction, or perhaps a little of both, nurses are an indispensable part of American health care and continue to practice with high standards. Their contribution is reflected in the unique services they provide in a variety of settings.

One thing is certain—nursing is a dynamic, vibrant field. In the real world, it may not exactly mirror the all-too-often romanticized picture portrayed in the media, but the opportunity to participate in a profession undergoing a dramatic transformation generates an exhilaration quite irreplaceable. The change is one of substance, involving much more than the shedding of the nurse's white cap and other traditional garb. Newer nursing roles have evolved, created by developments in scientific medicine, high tech innovation, reforms in the health care system, and more stringent standards in the education of nurses.

Modern nursing has come a long way since Florence Nightingale kept her nightly vigil, walking with her lamp through cramped hospital wards in Scutari. Or when the young, idealistic Louisa May Alcott endured her deprivations as a nurse in a Washington (DC) hospital during the Civil War. Or even when Lillian Wald's pioneering nurses of Henry Street climbed over New York City rooftops to reach their patients in the early 20th century.

Introduction

Although social conditions have markedly influenced the nurse's role and will continue to do so, nursing will always retain its two important core values of *caring* and *humanitarianism*. What has changed, however, is the dispelling of certain myths long held about the profession.

No longer do people think of nursing as a suitable occupation for young ladies to "merely fall back on after marriage and raising a family." Nurses today view their profession as a lifetime career, like their contemporaries in law, medicine, or business. They also have eradicated the handmaiden stereotype, and consider themselves full fledged colleagues of the physician working together in a complementary relationship. Furthermore, more men are being drawn to the field.

Interest in the profession has soared in recent years. More than ever, greater numbers of young people, and even the more mature, are flocking to colleges and universities to study nursing. You may be a high school student, a new graduate, or a "second careerist" eager to pursue challenges different from your previous experience. Keep in mind that no job in nursing need ever be static because you will be in a field that represents a career within a career.

Throughout your professional life, your goals will probably change. Perhaps you will begin as a staff nurse on a hospital's medical-surgical unit. In time, with the right preparation, guidance, and perseverance, you may want to advance to an oncology nurse specialist, transplant nurse coordinator, or a nurse practitioner; or you might aspire to become a faculty member, researcher, or a certified nurse-midwife. The opportunities are mind-boggling!

Although the direction you seek will depend, to a large extent, on your knowledge and skills, a big factor will be the innovations in health care yet to appear on the horizon. Predictions about nurses in the 21st century indicate that the greatest demand will be for those prepared for advanced clinical nursing practice, primary care in the community, and entrepreneurial activities.

Nursing: The Career of a Lifetime is a show and tell work, giving accurate and up-to-date information on everything you want to know about nursing. You will uncover something about its rich and enduring heritage, and discover the many present opportunities shared first hand by real life practicing nurses. You will learn what it takes to be a nurse, what educational program is best for you, where the challenging jobs are, how to move up on the career ladder, and how to position yourself as a professional person within your field and in American life.

This book will help you to determine how to invest in your future by becoming a professional nurse. Be assured—one of the most exciting adventures awaits you on your journey into nursing as a career.

Shirley H. Fondiller

Barbara J. Nerone

1

What's It All
About, Florence?

Because your profession is something you'll always have, you will
want to know something about its heritage, how nursing is defined,
and what it takes to achieve a successful and satisfying career.

The history of nursing is closely linked to the history of
women. Although men in the field are still a minority, they also
can claim strong historical roots that evolved during the monastic
movement following the birth of Christianity. In many cases, care
of the sick, helpless, and infirm became the permanent vocation of
large numbers of both men and women who joined religious orders.

Recorded accounts of ancient Greek life begin with the writings of Homer's *The Iliad* and *The Odyssey,* that nation's most sa-
cred works. Through Greek mythology, we discover the origins of
a people, as well as graphic descriptions of their health, illnesses,
and medical practices.

Fascinating tales are recounted about the ruling gods and god-
desses, and the magic of such names as Apollo, the patron of medicine and music, becomes familiar. During the 13th century B.C.,
Apollo's son Asclepios (known as Aesculapius in Rome), the god
of medicine, became famous as the architect of the exquisitely dec-
orated healing temples which were located in areas of natural
beauty, and fed by spring water.

These health resorts expanded into social and intellectual centers and drew not only the infirm but people who came to revel in the beauty of the surroundings. The popular health spas of today, found in many Western cultures, may be less elaborate and limited in function, but to some extent they can be viewed as vestiges of the early healing temples.

The daughters of Asclepios and his wife, Epione, carried on the family tradition of representing health in its various manifestations. Hygieia, as the goddess of health, personified miraculous all-healing herbs. Her sisters included Panacea, the restorer of health, Aegle, the "light of the sun," Meditrina, the preserver of health (probably the forerunner of the public health nurse), and Iaso, who represented the recovery from illness.

In the annals of Greek life, there emerges the important figure of Hippocrates (460–370 B.C.), who earned his title as the Father of Medicine. Hippocrates introduced the concept of rational or scientific medicine, in which he theorized that disease was not caused by spirits, demons, or gods but by the breaking of nature's laws. He perceived the physician's true art as assisting nature to produce a cure. His legacy to the medical profession appears prominently in the Hippocratic Oath, which contains ethical principles adopted later by modern nursing in the Florence Nightingale Pledge.

THE OLDEST ART AND THE YOUNGEST PROFESSION

Early Judeo-Christian teachings of love and brotherhood not only transformed the larger society but they set the foundation for organized nursing. During the Middle Ages, the Augustinian Sisters formed the first nursing order. Following the establishment of European medicine as a profession in the 13th century, the infamous witch-craze erupted with its main thrust on laywomen healers helping those afflicted with poverty and disease, and who were without physicians and hospitals.

These "wise women" or witches came from the lower classes and were often midwives traveling from village to village and home to home. They had a host of herbal remedies tested by many years of use, with some considered highly effective in modern pharmacology, such as digitalis for heart conditions and belladonna as an antispasmodic.

The healing practices of the witches became a threat to physicians, but even more so to the Catholic Church which catered to a ruling class that cultivated the university-prepared doctor. As an empiricist, the witch relied on her senses rather than faith or religious doctrine and practiced by trial and error as well as cause and effect. In a sense, her "magic" was the science of the times. The Church, in contrast, was anti-empirical.

Accused of such heinous acts as murder and poisoning, along with sexual crimes, the witches were fiercely attacked and burned at the stake in large numbers. Their cause also represented a political and class struggle. Although witch hunting eventually declined and death penalties were abolished in some European countries, a belief in the healing practices of witches persisted into the 18th century.

During the Renaissance Movement in the 1500s, the scientific method of inquiry was introduced and advances occurred in the medical profession with the growth of anatomical knowledge and its application to surgery. The Renaissance also created a split in the Church and led to the Protestant Reformation. Interest in religion and church support waned and monasteries closed, resulting in the "Dark Period" when hospitals became unsanitary places and nursing was performed by women like Dickens' notorious Sairy Gamp and Betsy Prig.

Perhaps no story has been told more often and more eloquently than that of Florence Nightingale, the founder of modern nursing. She earned her greatest recognition during the Crimean War, structuring nursing into an orderly work force. In 1860, she established the first school of nursing at St. Thomas Hospital in London, which operated as an entirely independent institution financed by the Nightingale Fund.

The school aimed to train hospital nurses, instruct them in the training of others, and prepare district nurses for the poor. Students went into the homes as well as the hospital and taught patients and families about maintaining and preserving their health.

Nightingale viewed nursing as a career and a calling, not a religious vocation. She expected students to have intelligence and impeccable morals and behavior. The opening of the Nightingale School represented not only a model to be replicated, but a new way of life for women throughout the world.

THE EARLY AMERICAN EXPERIENCE

In early America, the provision of medical care and nursing depended, to a large extent, upon the customs that the colonists brought with them from the homeland. The Pilgrim Fathers practiced a strict way of life, with the educated men in the community—the clergy, school teachers, or governors—assuming the role of the physician. At the same time, superstition abounded with Indian folklore intermingled with prayer in treating disease.

As a function of the religious community, nursing in the New World involved devoted service and "saving souls." Since hospitals developed slowly in the thirteen colonies, relatives or friends became the caregivers. In the early 16th century, the poor who became sick, however, were sent to almshouses that gradually evolved into separate municipal hospitals.

Founded by physicians in 1751, the Pennsylvania Hospital in Philadelphia (later changed to Pennsylvania General Hospital) was the first institution in the United States to operate solely for the curative care of the sick. Conditions there were crude, with nursing provided by servant women who often worked on the wards housing the insane. The most prominent physician of the time was Benjamin Rush, known for his care of the mentally ill.

The establishment of the American Medical Association in 1847 was an important step in advancing the science of medicine. But it was not until 1911 that significant reform in medical education was initiated, following a study sponsored by the Carnegie Foundation and conducted by Abraham Flexner. During that period when nursing was just a fledgling profession, it too was struggling to upgrade its educational standards and eliminate the unquestionable practices of unqualified women calling themselves "nurses."

The 20th century saw the rapid growth of nursing and its assimilation into American society. The movement, however, which had begun earlier was precipitated by several factors that coalesced to form the foundation of organized nursing.

PRELUDE TO ORGANIZED NURSING

The advent of the Industrial Revolution, rising immigration, scientific innovations, and urbanization transformed American life during the 1800s. Prior to the Civil War, a spirit of volunteerism was pervasive, created by the benevolence of women—called the "charitable impulse"—to the humanitarian concerns of the period.

Volunteerism proved to be a significant development because it expanded the competence of women and resulted in the acceptance, for the first time, of those who worked (without pay) outside the home. Volunteers in the Ladies Aid Societies that sprung up at the outset of the Civil War in April 1861, included nurses and other women who gave direct services—"comforts and necessities"—to the soldiers at the front. Dorothea Dix, a longtime spokesperson for the mentally ill, was appointed Superintendent of Female Nurses of the Union Army.

The war drew over 2,000 women from the North and South, who served as nurses in military hospitals and on hospital ships, trains, and wagons. The haunting recollections of Louisa May Alcott in her *Hospital Sketches*, offer her firsthand account as a volunteer nurse assigned to Washington's (DC) Union Hotel Hospital. Another volunteer nurse was the poet Walt Whitman, who eloquently recorded in his journal his readings to the wounded, writing letters for them, and assisting with dressings and operations.

And who can forget the courageous and dedicated black nurse, Harriet Tubman, better known for escorting thousands of slaves to freedom in the underground railroad? She treated many Union soldiers successfully with her special brew concocted from a water lily, a plant common to her native Maryland.

The humanitarian values of nurses, and their love of country, have sustained them through many wars. Some like Clarissa (Clara) Barton, who founded the American Red Cross and was the first

5

woman volunteer to take to the battlefield in the Civil War, remain enduring heroines in nursing's heritage. Her heroism, along with others, set the stage for the beginning of the modern nursing movement in the United States.

THE MODERN NURSING MOVEMENT

The Civil War, and its aftermath, generated high interest in nursing education, which led to the simultaneous appearance of three schools of nursing in the early 1870s. The famous trio consisted of the Bellevue Training School in New York City, Connecticut Training School in New Haven, and the Boston Training School (later changed to the Massachusetts General Hospital School of Nursing).

Although the intent was to create the schools independent of hospital control, as proposed in the Nightingale model, they were soon absorbed by the parent institution because of a lack of funding. Once established, the apprentice system of preparing nurses in hospital diploma programs became the recognized pattern.

Almost from the beginning, there existed a built-in weakness since many hospitals soon discovered that schools could be established to serve their needs, including a free source of labor. Thus, the school's real function was one of service rather than education. It would be many decades before the profession's educational system would undergo any major change.

The late 19th century proved to be a fertile period for the budding profession. Influenced by the work of Florence Nightingale and progressive British nurses like Ethel Manson Fenwick, a group of courageous women assembled during the Chicago World's Fair in 1893 to establish the first national nursing association in the United States. The American Society of Superintendents of Training Schools for Nurses (renamed the National League of Nursing Education in 1912) aimed to establish and maintain a universal standard of education.

The Society's efforts led to the founding of the Nurses Associated Alumnae of the United States and Canada in 1896 (renamed the American Nurses Association in 1911). The alumnae organization was designed to strengthen the union of the existing affiliates and accommodate the needs of practicing nurses. Eventually, these groups evolved into state nursing associations.

In 1899, Teachers College, Columbia University, became the first institution of higher learning to concern itself with nursing education. It introduced a course in hospital economics, an event of some import because it placed nursing within collegiate education and was a giant step toward advancing the profession.

At the turn of the century, women's clubs, churches, charity organizations, settlement houses, health departments, and hospitals were hiring nurses to care for the sick. Training schools had proliferated by this time, which created some concern since a flagrant disregard for standards soon became apparent. The establishment of the national nursing organizations reflected an effort of the profession to regulate its practice and ensure the public's safety and welfare.

In the early 1900s, nursing leaders began a drive toward state registration to meet the need for legally approved standards. The movement gained momentum through the new *American Journal of Nursing* and the burgeoning state associations. Nursing practice acts were enacted to define professional practice.

Over the years, the dramatic changes in nursing and health care, plus the ambiguity in the laws among the states, stimulated in-depth review. During the mid-1970s, New York State became the first jurisdiction in the nation to revise its nursing practice act, which distinguished between nursing and medical practice, and acknowledged nursing as an autonomous profession.

A significant period in nursing's development occurred at the outset of World War II and the decades to follow. In 1943, the profession spawned one of its greatest recruitment efforts through a government-sponsored campaign to meet the nation's need for nurses. Thousands of young people flocked to nursing schools to sign up for the Cadet Nurse Corps.

Around that time, nursing leaders initiated a study to explore the possibility of consolidating the number of national groups that had sprung up over the years. In the early 1950s, a major restructuring took place, in which five organizations were assimilated into the American Nurses Association (ANA) and the new National League for Nursing (NLN).

Postwar America began to undergo a radical transformation in the nature and delivery of health care services. Organized medicine moved rapidly toward specialization and hospital reorganization followed. Recovery rooms and intensive care units were increasingly visible, along with new groups of health workers. The age of technology arrived, and erupted full blown within a couple of decades.

On the nursing scene, innovative practices were well underway in the 1970s, with nurse practitioners and clinical nurse specialists representing a new breed in the field. The rise of specialization led to the formation of national organizations, reaching the phenomenal number of almost 100 by 1990! It wasn't long before a host of nursing journals came on the coattails of their respective specialty groups.

THE MOVERS AND SHAKERS— WHO WERE THEY?

No history would be complete without mentioning some of the people who fostered the advancement of the nursing profession. As nursing developed, its direction paralleled the events in the larger society. Nurses were part of the action, pitching in with all their know-how to improve the standards of health care and quality of life.

To honor those nurses whose achievements significantly affected the profession, the ANA inaugurated the Nursing Hall of Fame during the nation's bicentennial in 1976. From a list of more than 100 names, it selected fifteen charter members to be immortalized.

Included among the first group was Lillian Wald, credited as the founder of public health nursing (see Figure 1.1). With her cadre of Henry Street nurses, they carried the torch at the turn of the century to help poor and sick immigrant families on New York City's lower east side.

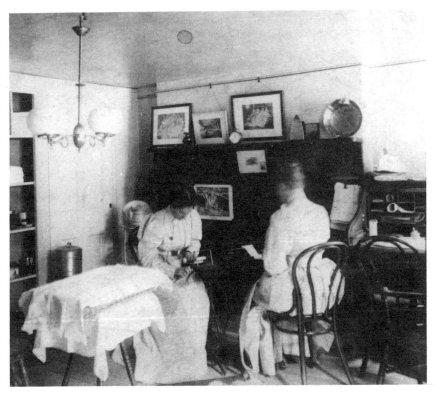

Figure 1.1 Lillian Wald (left) and Mary Brewster, founders of the New York Visiting Nurse Service, roll bandages in their original tenement apartment on Jefferson Street, about 1894. (Courtesy of Visiting Nurse Service of New York.)

One of Henry Street's most distinguished alumnae was Annie Goodrich, who became dean and professor at Yale, which instituted the first experimental university-based school of nursing in 1923. Another Henry Street nurse was the remarkable Lavinia Dock, a social activist whose prolific writings aimed to move nursing forward, as well as advance the cause of woman's suffrage.

Among the profession's illustrious leaders was Mary Breckinridge, a nurse-midwife who introduced the first modern rural comprehensive health care system in the United States. As the founder of the Frontier Nursing Service at Wendover, Kentucky, in 1928, she and her staff became known as the "Nurses on Horseback," providing nursing and midwifery services 24 hours a day.

Remembered as one of nursing's great reformers in women's health, the charismatic and controversial Margaret Sanger pioneered the American birth control movement. In 1942, she founded Planned Parenthood of America, and ten years later the International Planned Parenthood Foundation.

Too numerous to cite, nursing's leaders of yesteryear have left their mark. Some have been dramatized in film and television stories, while others appear in biographical works and the growing body of literature by nurse historians.

Nursing today has its own movers and shakers who aptly follow in the tradition of their gallant forebears. They perform admirably in various practice settings, educational institutions, research, professional organizations, and a variety of other areas. The recent growth of nursing centers, managed and controlled by nurses, represents one of the most exciting trends in the profession. It also illustrates how nursing has come full circle in strengthening its early roots in the community while moving vigorously into the 21st century.

2

What It Takes to Be a Nurse

In determining whether nursing might be the career for you, consider carefully what there is about the profession that particularly attracts you. You could be right on target as to what being a nurse is really like. Then again, your perceptions may be a little fuzzy, or just plain wrong.

For example, if you think that the program of study will be comparatively easy, or even a lark, forget it! Nursing is a rigorous discipline, generating satisfaction and self-discovery in the bright, creative person. Another myth is that becoming a nurse can be a stepping stone to the medical profession. The fact is that few nurses go into medicine. Among those who wish to pursue a doctorate eventually, most earn the degree in their own field.

WHAT IS THE NATURE OF NURSING?

Just as there are many reasons that inspire people to enter the profession, various definitions have evolved through the years describing the nature of the work. The derivation of the word *nursing* can be traced to the Latin *nutrice* meaning "to nourish." *Nutrix* also came from the Latin, which translated into "nursing mother." Gradually, the concept broadened to include women caring for young children.

By the 16th century, nursing expanded to waiting upon or tending the ill. Another dimension was added to the term in the 1800s, with the *training* of those who cared for the sick.

Although nurturing is a value associated with modern nursing, its earlier roots show a closer relationship to education. In the rearing of the young in European cultures, the nursemaid or governess was a prominent figure in the role of the child-nurse. Nurturing, however, has remained an important component of nursing in delivering compassionate care.

Over a hundred years ago, Florence Nightingale described nursing within a clean, well-ventilated room and quiet environment to help patients in their recovery. She emphasized the independent functions of the nurse, which included preventive care along with the safety and comfort of the person.

In American nursing, Virginia Henderson was one of the first nurses to offer her interpretation which has become a classic in the profession. Three decades ago, she defined nursing as:

> The unique function of the nurse is to assist the individual, sick or well, in the performance of those activities contributing to health or its recovery (or to peaceful death) that he would perform unaided if he had the necessary strength, will, or knowledge, and to do this in such a way as to help him gain independence as rapidly as possible.

Subsequently, other definitions have sprung up, but all reflect the goals of health promotion, health maintenance and restoration, and care of the dying. Simply stated, nursing has been characterized as caring for a sick or disabled person, or one unable to provide for their own basic needs.

In a more contemporary view, the definition has been expanded to emphasize care of the "whole" person, or holistic care, which stresses wellness rather than describing health in relation to diseases. Many nurses refer to health recipients as clients rather than patients since the focus is on the individual's responsibility for his or her own health habits. The role of nurses as advocates for persons in their care is to assist them in their own actions and encourage their participation in making informed decisions.

WHY BE A NURSE?

You now have a clearer idea of how nursing is defined. You may still wonder about the number of titles ascribed to people working in the field. What's the difference between a registered nurse (RN) and a licensed practical nurse (LPN)? Who are nurse practitioners? Nurse-Midwives? Are they nurses, too? And what about nursing assistants or nurses aides?

Have patience—at least for a while. All your questions will be answered eventually. You will discover how the performance of nurses fits the title they have earned, whether it's a staff nurse, nurse manager, clinical nurse specialist, or even a vice president for nursing.

For the moment, however, your concern is why you think nursing might be *the* career for you. Undoubtedly, you already realize that the variability of human beings in determining a particular choice makes it difficult, perhaps even impossible, to pinpoint the predominant factors that influence a career decision.

Whatever your reasons, one constant remains—the opportunity to grow as a person and a professional. If you are someone who likes the independence of working or living in different parts of the nation, then pick your spot. Or, if you have a yen for far off lands and exotic cultures, you might want to consider the Peace Corps or Project Hope.

Exciting challenges await those who sign up with the armed forces. Will it be the army, navy, or air force nurse corps? Military nursing offers great perks that include formal schooling, overseas assignments, and financial security.

To assist you in making your decision, listen to some of the following thoughts expressed by nurses practicing in the field. See if their reasons for going into nursing match your own.

For Joyce Keeler, neonatal and transport nurse at University of California Medical Center in Los Angeles, her first exposure to nursing came through a little Golden Book called *Nurse*

Nancy. "I was only five years old but I was able to read about the nurse who helped her brother when he was stung by a bee!" declares Keeler. "And ever since I wanted to be a nurse so I could help people."

Surprisingly, books about nursing targeted to a young audience have left their mark on many a prospective nurse. The story line might be a bit unrealistic and the plot over dramatized, but somehow the idea of the caring, nurturing heroine always comes through.

For over two decades, Helen Wells' books on *Cherry Ames,* covering the youthful RN in a variety of jobs and places, became a familiar name in almost every American household. As far back as World War II, Wells (who was not a nurse) initiated her series. Another popular heroine of the same period was the ubiquitous *Sue Barton.*

Keeler admits the fictional Nancy was an early influence, since the work lit a spark in her. By the time she reached her teens, she was well into reading biographies about "real" nurses like Clara Barton. "During Vietnam, I wanted to be a *MASH* (Mobile Army Surgical Hospital) nurse but was too young," she recalls. "So, there was never a question about what career I wanted."

Some nurses like Kristine Hunt, a hospice/oncology practitioner at Presbyterian Hospital in Charlotte, North Carolina, come from a background having a parent or family relative as a nurse. "My grandmother was an old time practical nurse and my older sister a licensed practical nurse," reports Hunt. "I was born being altruistic. My mother says I was a 40-year-old infant!"

A common reason for someone seeking a career in nursing is the impact of an earlier experience with illness or hospitalization. Linda Anderson, the chief manager of the Arthritic Care Center at Baptist Hospital in Nashville, Tennessee, suffered a serious burn as a youngster. She described the nurses who cared for her as "wonderful." She also was impressed by the public health nurse in the school in her rural community. "I thought she was a very special person."

When Keith Bradkowski worked at other jobs prior to nursing, he knew that he wanted a career change. "I looked at a

14

number of the health professions including medical school, and realized that nursing was in the forefront of health care delivery," states Bradkowski. Beginning as a staff nurse and later a clinical specialist in psychiatric/mental health nursing, he recently advanced to the position of administrative director of patient care services at Santa Monica-UCLA Medical Center (see Figure 2.1).

Many nurses get their first taste of the profession as hospital candy stripers or nursing assistants when in high school. Others, however, cannot point to any single factor that perked their interest in nursing. Perhaps you fit into this category. Maybe it is just a gut feeling.

"I had no nurse role model growing up," says Joanna Boatman, a charge nurse at Virginia Mason Hospital in Seattle, Washington. "But I always wanted to be a nurse."

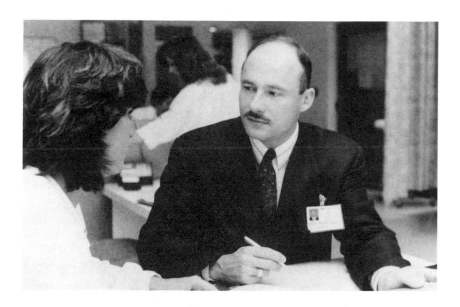

Figure 2.1 Keith Bradkowski, shown with nurse colleague, at Santa Monica-UCLA Medical Center.

WHAT DOES IT TAKE?

When it comes to determining what it takes to be a nurse, it's surprising that some of the old myths haven't gone out with high button shoes! A few years ago, an astute nurse remarked that equating nursing with bedpan carrying was like comparing parenting with changing diapers. Mary Mallison, the editor of the *American Journal of Nursing* at the time, commented on the nurse's analogy: "A lot of nursing resembles the best kind of parenting," she said. "Supporting people until they can help themselves, and strengthening their belief in themselves."*

Perhaps you're wondering if nursing seeks a certain type of person to enter its ranks. Unquestionably, such traits as intelligence, perseverance, and flexibility are desirable in any profession. In nursing, however, additional characteristics have taken on increasing importance in the changing health care scene.

Dramatic medical and technological advances have generated new kinds of roles for nurses, calling for well-developed communication skills and risk taking behaviors. Just look at the nurse practitioner movement and the clinical impact these nurses are having in hospitals and in the community. The list goes on and on with other models springing up as nurses strive to improve patient care.

As to what you really need to make a *good* nurse, it would be a bit foolhardy to lay claim to a specific stereotypical mold. After all, who can identify the person that will become the *perfect* doctor, attorney, or business executive? Nevertheless, you may be able to detect certain commonalities among professional nurses that loom much larger than their differences. Following are the thoughts of some of these nurses as they share their views:

Dyan Aretakis, a family nurse practitioner and project director at University of Virginia in Charlottesville, considers a "well developed ego and a good sense of self" a big plus in nursing. What she ranks highest, however, are "incredible person skills. You must

* Mallison, M. (1986) "Letter to a high school counselor." *American Journal of Nursing*, 86(5):517.

16

be enthusiastic and engaging," she declares. "Then you can heal people by dramatically affecting how they are coping."

There's no question that nursing is a people business. Part of the excitement of being in the field is providing your services to individuals from different walks of life, and of ages ranging from the cradle to the very old. "The ability to work with all kinds of people requires a lot of compassion," claims Margaret Moran, a staff nurse with the Visiting Nurse Association of Eastern Montgomery County in Willow Park, Pennsylvania. She adds that the nurse "must think and act quickly with sound judgment."

Well accepted as a core value in nursing, compassion is viewed by many nurses as having the capacity to meet people as they are and to put their needs above everything else. Some even go so far as to say that nurses must be able to "see through the eyes of their patients and walk in their shoes."

Compassion is also at the top of the list of qualities cited by Mary Jo Modica, a transplant nurse manager at Ohio State University Medical Center in Columbus. Equally important, she notes, are commitment and motivation. "You need to be a patient/family advocate first and foremost."

Modica points out that a nurse has to juggle many tasks at once, which means setting priorities in nursing care plans. "You have to know how to communicate with patients as well as with physicians and other groups."

Working as a pediatric nurse practitioner at Children's National Medical Center in Washington (DC), Catherine Ernsthausen echoes many of the thoughts already expressed. "I think there are many qualities a nurse should have, including problem-solving skills, patience, and energy."

Thomas Steeves' perception of what it takes to be a nurse is "a sense of calling." A staff/charge nurse at Abbott Northwestern Hospital in Minneapolis, Minnesota, he believes that in addition to being assertive and humble, the most desirable characteristics are "intelligence and a good heart, which make for the best in today's technological environment."

* * *

The preceding views appear to be representative of most professional nurses. Think about them and then explore your own needs. Keep in mind, however, that individual differences exist in every field, which should enrich rather than deter the discipline. After all, you will want to pursue a career in which you can be free to learn, to express yourself, and to share and challenge ideas with colleagues in practice, the classroom, and in other settings.

Long ago, Nightingale described nursing as "the finest of the fine arts." It is a giving profession, and one whose returns are immeasurable. Yet, what greater reward can there be than making a difference in the lives of people, helping and supporting them through the continuum of health. That's what nursing is all about!

3

The Employment Arena:
What Are Your Prospects?

It is difficult to believe that there are more than two million registered nurses in the United States, with over 80 percent employed!
Two thirds of this large contingent work in hospitals. An increasing
number, however, is shifting to long-term care, home health care,
ambulatory and school-based clinics, health maintenance organizations, and community nursing centers.

Nurses also teach in schools of nursing, serve in executive positions, conduct research, and share joint practices with other nurses
or physicians. In addition, opportunities flourish in the military
and in government service. Several international agencies sponsor
nurses for overseas assignments that may include assisting developing nations with their health programs.

All these options may seem a bit overwhelming, but they only
enhance nursing's appeal as an exciting career. Just look at the
growth of enrollments in college and university nursing programs.
According to a 1994 survey by the National League for Nursing,
close to one fourth of newly licensed nurses indicated that they had
a college degree in another field prior to their nursing education.

You undoubtedly want to know more about the nature of the
profession's workforce. Before piquing your interest further, however, it might be helpful to define as simply as possible the two

umbrella categories associated with nursing since marked differences exist between the registered nurse (RN) and the licensed practical nurse (LPN) or licensed vocational nurse (LVN).

In Chapter 7 you will find more information about the education and expectations of the RN and the LPN/LVN. In the meantime, here are the two groups broadly defined:

> A registered nurse is a licensed, independent health care provider legally responsible for his or her own practice. To be eligible for licensure, a person must have graduated from a state approved school of nursing, and passed the registered nurse licensing examination.

> A licensed practical nurse or licensed vocational nurse is a person who has graduated from a state approved school of practical nursing and has passed the state board examination for practical nursing.

Within the profession, multiculturalism and ethnic diversity have long been championed. In light of the improved economic climate, business and entrepreneurial opportunities, and satisfaction on the job, more men are being drawn to nursing. Although the majority of nurses are women, the number of male graduates has almost doubled in the last few years.

A 1992 report of the *National Sample Survey of Registered Nurses* reveals that 4.0 percent of employed nurses are men. The same source also provides data on ethnic-racial background, with 91.1 percent of RNs representing Whites/non-Hispanic, 4.0 percent Blacks, 3.4 percent Asians/Islanders, 1.4 percent Hispanics, and 0.4 percent American Indians/Alaskans.

Among full-time employees, baccalaureate graduates constitute the largest number; 31 percent of nurses work part time. As to marital status, almost three-fourths of actively practicing RNs are married, 16.5 percent divorced, separated, or widowed, and 11.1 percent have never married.

Will there be a job for me? This is an obvious question, but important when considering a particular career choice. Your desire to enter nursing or perhaps teaching, journalism, or some other profession may be only a dream right now, but it is one that you will want to convert into reality and bring you long-term fulfillment. Your main concern in following a certain course is to make your decision thoughtfully. That means getting the big picture and not just a bird's-eye view of the field you wish to pursue.

With nursing as your potential goal, you will need to have at your fingertips the facts and figures about the present job market. Even more critical are the changes anticipated in health care in the years ahead, along with the employment requirements and practices expected of professional nurses. Some of the newer nursing roles are already quite visible in ambulatory settings and in the community. Table 3.1, which compares data on places of employment in 1992 and 1988, reflects trends over a four-year period.

You're probably aware of the much publicized nursing shortage of the 1980s, which abated by the 1990s. In recent times,

TABLE 3.1   Places of Employment of Registered Nurses

	1992 Estimated Percent	1988 Estimated Percent
Ambulatory Care Setting MD Practices, HMOS Group Practice, Nurse-Based Practices, Other Ambulatory Settings	7.8	7.7
Community/Public Health Setting	9.7	6.8
Hospital	66.5	67.9
Nursing Education	2.0	1.8
Nursing Home/Extended Care Facility	7.0	6.6
Occupational Health	2.7	1.3
Student Health Service	2.7	2.9
Other	3.0	3.6
Not Known	.2	—

Source: Moses, Evelyn B. *The Registered Nurse Population.* National Sample Survey, DHHS Division of Nursing, 1988, 1992.

however, a dramatic reversal has occurred with a general downward trend in hospital employment. Nevertheless, it's a good idea to keep in mind that all fields tend to go through cycles of ups and downs created by a variety of factors. Although nursing leaders are alerted to these developments, they recognize that there always will be a need for nurses since people require the care of well qualified professionals. Nursing roles may undergo change, but the basic values of caring and compassion remain constant.

Be assured that job prospects of newly licensed nurses are excellent. In NLN's 1994 survey of this group, 90 percent indicated that they found employment within three months of graduation, and are continuing in the same position. Among these nurses, 81 percent work in hospitals, beginning at the staff level. Large numbers are located on medical/surgical units or intensive care units. This fact supports the notion by experts that critical care is becoming the main focus of acute care hospitals.

On the salary front, the news is good. In 1992, the average annual rate for beginning nurses was $28,586 and $37,738 for those more experienced. More recently, an upswing in salaries has occurred for the new RN averaging $29,384, although regional variations exist. When considering salary in the general nursing population, employers assess such factors as the type and requirements of the position along with the credentials and experience of the nurse.

The kinds of work opportunities open to nurses cover a wide range. Perhaps your choice in time will be on an inpatient unit of a hospital or medical center. Or how about the outpatient area where you can do ambulatory nursing? Maybe you will be captivated by the thought of nursing in the community, which is said to be *the* place of the future.

That decision may seem like a long way off but it is something to think about as you move along in your nursing program. Even then, you may change your mind several times! Nursing students are known to enjoy one clinical rotation after another, with the last one almost always the favorite—at least for the moment. By the end of the course, however, you will have a good idea of the next step in launching your new career.

Since most RNs begin in staff nurse positions in hospitals, you will want to learn more about these institutions. How are they organized? Who are the key players and decision makers? What about the patterns of nursing care? And what kinds of challenges await nurses in this fascinating world that seems to take on a life of its own?

If you worked as a candy striper or nurse's aide, or spent time in a hospital as a visitor or patient, then you already have formed some definite impressions. Yet, the changing climate within facilities has greatly altered the delivery of patient services. Restructuring, reorganizing, and re-engineering have become the buzzwords of the nineties. Attempting to seek better and less costly ways to provide care, administrators have turned to alternative methods. Therefore, in cluing you in on the latest trends and developments affecting the modern hospital, you will acquire fresh insights about nursing in institutions long considered the mainstay of the American health care system.

THE MODERN HOSPITAL: WHAT YOU NEED TO KNOW

Hospitals have experienced a marked decline in census over the past decade, which can be attributed to a number of factors. To cut down on expensive hospitalization, many procedures have been successfully performed in the outpatient department, where one-day surgery has become almost commonplace.

Another effort to make hospital care more cost effective has been the introduction of prospective payment systems since the early 1980s. Under this arrangement, the federal government, which provides funding to hospitals for Medicare and Medicaid patients, has designated a predetermined length of stay (making it shorter) according to the diagnosis-related group (DRG) in which the person has been categorized. As a result, patients have been discharged more rapidly, and often require complex and highly technological care in the home. DRGs, however, have reduced hospital utilization.

An important factor affecting hospital stays is the growing popularity of health maintenance organizations (HMOs). The HMO represents one type of managed care, a term you have been hearing a lot about in discussions of health care reform. It combines the delivery of full health services into one system involving a fixed prepaid fee to members. These services may be provided in facilities owned by the HMO, generally for ambulatory care, or through contract with other hospitals.

In the United States, hospitals have become big business, well on the track to becoming large corporate entities nationwide. What was once a collection of single institutions, independently run, moderate in size, and comprised of a simplified organizational structure has become the exception rather than the rule.

The push has been toward the acquisition or merging of the smaller hospital into a multi-institutional system. This means that there may be two or more hospitals owned, leased, sponsored, or contract managed by a central organization. Between 1980 and 1992, the health care industry averaged about 16 mergers a year.

There are economic advantages to this trend in regard to shared purchasing of material resources and technology, the use of technical and management staff, and joint programming and activities. Above all, the prime goal is to improve access to care and the delivery of patient services. You may already be familiar with such names as Hospital Corporation of America (HCA), American International (AMI), or Humana.

From the early 1980s to 1990, almost 500 hospitals closed, due mainly to financial pressures and changing health care practices. In 1994, close to 6,000 hospitals were listed in the nation, with about a fifth classified as teaching institutions. Hospitals of this variety are generally in medical centers having more than 400 beds. They offer accredited medical residency programs, in which medical students and/or resident and specialty fellows are taught. In addition, they serve as clinical learning sites for nursing students.

Large medical centers that house one thousand or more patients are usually combined teaching and research facilities that offer a variety of tertiary (acute care) services. Most are referred to as academic health centers, encompassing schools in the health professions, such as medicine and nursing. Some teaching hospitals are also trauma centers, federally designated to treat the injured.

Hospitals differ in size, type, location, and ownership. They can vary from 25 to more than 2,000 beds. The two main groups in relation to size are the short-term general facility, which averages 160 beds, and long-term hospitals averaging 900 beds. Among these institutions, the most common type has been the voluntary, general, short-term, not-for-profit hospital. This category includes the larger teaching institution as well as the smaller, family-like community hospital.

Government hospitals represent a dominant group involved in delivering health care services. Did you know that the Veterans Administration operates the largest centrally directed hospital and clinic system? Another government agency is the Indian Health Service, which oversees hospitals, health centers, and satellite health clinics for Native Americans and Alaskan Natives.

As you can see, there is no dearth of hospitals and they all require the services of nurses. Besides the general hospital, there are public institutions including municipal and state facilities. In addition, many separate specialized hospitals exist for women and infants, rehabilitation centers, eye and ear infirmaries, psychiatric institutions, and a host of other facilities.

All types of hospitals are licensed by the state and have to maintain minimum standards prescribed by the licensing authority. You should be aware, however, that higher standards are fostered through voluntary accreditation by the Joint Commission on Accreditation of Healthcare Organizations (JCAHO). With the aim of indicating excellence in patient care, JCAHO's stringent standards measure hospital efficiency, professional performance (including nursing), and facilities.

CHANGING STRUCTURES AND STYLES

The way a hospital is organized in its administrative hierarchy as well as the physical layout of the various units can tell you a lot about that institution. The experts say that it all depends on the philosophy of the institution. Fortunately, centralized, standardized, and top-down organizations that focused on sameness and efficiency have surrendered increasingly to decentralized approaches throughout the system.

On nursing (clinical) units where decentralization has occurred, creative and joint planning evolves and innovations follow. Under participatory management where communication flows up and down and nurses contribute to the decision-making process in the care of their patients, nurses derive great satisfaction at the staff level. This type of environment is particularly important for new RNs to consider when exploring job opportunities.

As part of the corporate world, hospitals are experiencing increased competition and therefore attempting to bring new structures and management styles to the workplace. Long-time bureaucracies are beginning to give way to more democratic approaches. Some hospitals have formed matrix models, in which nurses, health systems staff, and other health professionals are grouped around special projects or tasks.

Although hospitals vary in physical structure from a one-level building to a high rise, commonalities exist in the general hospital. Most facilities house clinical units for patients, operating rooms and post anesthesia recovery suites, emergency departments, and critical care or intensive care units (ICUs). In addition, there are diagnostic and treatment units, laboratories, radiology departments, pharmacies, social services, and physicians' offices in some hospitals. Most institutions provide dietary and food services, housekeeping and laundry service, maintenance, storage, and other nonclinical services. You will also find conference rooms and classrooms as well as gift shops and waiting rooms for visitors.

At the helm of the hospital is the administrator, who may also hold the title of president or chief executive officer. This individual is directly responsible to a governing board of trustees. The administrative section usually includes the admissions office, and the various departments or offices dealing with personnel, business affairs, public relations, and medical records. The hospital administrator, the chief of the medical staff (or physician-in-chief), and the chief fiscal officer have comparable lines of authority in most institutions (see Figure 3.1).

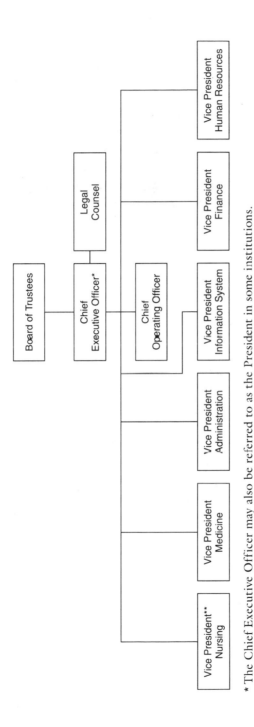

* The Chief Executive Officer may also be referred to as the President in some institutions.
** The title of Vice President varies from institution to institution and may be referred to as Associate Director.

Figure 3.1 Organizational Chart of a Traditional Medical Center.

The internal redesign of hospitals appears to be an ongoing process. Progressive administrators realize that the ambience of a facility is greatly influenced by its physical appearance. Happily gone in most places is the large ward with the sterile looking white walls and rows of old iron beds lined up side by side.

Cheerful wallpaper or pastel colors now decorate the clinical units where patients' rooms project a modern, homey look in spite of the electronic equipment. There is an increasing presence of computer terminals at the bedside, as well. On some units, creative arrangements have been instituted to promote a closeness between patients and the staff. One example is known as the quad system, in which every person's room becomes part of a semicircle around the nurses' station where RNs and physicians do their charts and record keeping.

STREAMLINING NURSING SERVICES

Just as hospitals and medical centers have taken on a new look, nursing services have undergone changes in delivery patterns. One reason is the kind of health problems facing the American public. Breakthroughs produced by medical research and advances in surgery have succeeded in either shortening the length of hospital stays or eliminating them completely. Although communicable diseases such as diphtheria and smallpox are long gone, other serious infectious illnesses have appeared on the health care scene in the form of HIV and AIDS, for example.

Over the years, nursing care has evolved from what was once the case method or private nursing to the present case management approach. Just look at an old mystery movie, or peruse a Mary Roberts Rinehart (she was an RN) novel, and you're bound to find a private duty nurse as one of the main characters. In the traditional sense, the private nurse has become more of a rarity since the advent of recovery rooms and ICUs.

Functional nursing was the next model to be introduced but it generated little satisfaction. Much fragmentation occurred since nurses performed only part of the care and no one was accountable. When team nursing followed, problems continued since the

RN supervised a group of lesser prepared workers and the patients could not differentiate professional nurses from other personnel.

During the 1970s, forward-looking hospitals initiated primary nursing, an approach in which the RN is accountable for an individual patient's care plan during a 24-hour period throughout a hospital stay. The primary nurse (a minimum of a baccalaureate is recommended) has direct contact with the patient's family, significant others, and members of the health team with whom cooperative planning occurs for total care and continuity. An associate nurse takes over when the primary nurse is off duty, but the latter has around-the-clock responsibility for his or her patients.

As an extension of primary nursing, case management has become a popular delivery model in recent years. It incorporates a broader view linking the nurse with a case-specific physician in collaborating on certain case types within DRGs. Specific plans, known as critical pathways, guide the case management team from even before the patient's admission through the course of hospitalization and into post-discharge care in the community. The pathways indicate events that must occur each day to achieve the proper length of stay. Through case management, nurses are in a key position to manage the costs and quality of health care.

During the 1980s, another model called differentiated nursing practice was launched, with the purpose of distinguishing professional (baccalaureate) and technical (associate degree or diploma) roles from the present single role of the RN. This pattern first appeared in the Midwest but it has caught on in some facilities in other regions.

In some hospitals where staffing of professional nurses is limited, a staff RN will team up with a licensed practical or vocational nurse to care for the same patients. The term "Partners-in-Practice" has been applied to this arrangement, in which the registered nurse is responsible for managing the plan of care. Both workers, however, assume accountability for the tasks distributed between them.

Not every hospital utilizes the same approach to nursing care. How RNs deliver their services in a particular facility is based on several considerations, such as the complement and qualifications of staff, the number of patients, and the autonomy given to practice in the manner that nurses have been taught. You can be sure that new modes will surface from time to time according to the changing needs of patients.

Who Are the Nurses?

As noted earlier, today's patients are different from those of yesteryear, and so it is not surprising that new drugs, therapies, and technologies have all mandated radical changes in nursing care.

The nursing service within a hospital is an impressive part of the organization since it is the largest individual department, consisting of more than half of the total number of employees. The members not only carry out unique functions, but they have specific titles that designate status within the institution. So, if someone asks— *What's in a name,* you would be quite right in saying—*More than you think in the hospital world!*

The first-level position for RNs is general duty or staff nurse. As a staff nurse, your job would be to complement the physician's treatment regimen and develop and implement a plan of care tailored to each patient's condition. You would give direct hands-on care and provide some health teaching and counseling to patients and their support people.

In their practice, staff nurses apply the nursing process as a problem-solving approach, which is the basis of nursing. Although many RNs have opportunities to move up to managerial posts, some prefer to remain in general duty because of the close contact with their patients.

On nursing units, the nurse manager has replaced the traditional head nurse in many facilities, giving the role broader scope and responsibility. First-line managers may also be called clinical directors or patient care coordinators. Their prime functions are to carry out administrative duties, assure quality in nursing practice, and help staff in making decisions. At this level, the work may be shared with other nurses serving as assistants or associates.

It is good to remember that considerable variation exists not only in titles but in positions within the nursing service department. A major factor is the size of the facility. Some hospitals continue to employ middle managers or supervisors, who represent the next rung of the nursing ladder. The role is ill defined but, in general, the supervisor oversees several clinical units that may be grouped according to location or specialty.

The highest position in the nursing hierarchy belongs to the nurse executive, who may be referred to as the director of nursing, director of nursing service, chief nurse, or nurse administrator. If the person is viewed as part of the top eschelons of hospital administration, then his or her title may be vice-president of nursing, or assistant or associate administrator.

In academic health centers, some nurse executives hold joint appointments as deans or associate deans of college or university nursing programs. This practice aims to draw nursing service and nursing education closer together. The same principle applies to clinical specialists and nurse practitioners who work in the hospital or community while holding faculty appointments.

A hospital position requiring up-to-date knowledge is the staff development instructor or coordinator. As a nurse educator, this person develops learning activities based on the needs of the staff to enhance their job performance. Orientation, in-service education, and continuing education comprise the three facets of staff development.

Other positions for RNs that you will find in some hospitals are those of nurse researcher and nurse epidemiologist or infection control nurse. Also visible, particularly in the larger medical center, are nurses in advanced practice, such as clinical nurse specialists, nurse practitioners, certified nurse-midwives, and certified nurse anesthetists.

The smooth running of a nursing unit requires the services of clerical and well-trained support personnel. Nursing assistants, sometimes referred to as aides, orderlies, or attendants perform nonclinical tasks, such as transporting, fetching, message taking, carrying, and other similar activities often left to the nurse. In this way, RNs are free to devote their skills to the nursing care of patients.

Another recent addition to the corporate scene is that of the nurse intrapreneur. You might be more familiar with the word entrepreneur, which refers to a person who organizes and manages some type of business and assumes any risk related to profit. Later, you will learn more about nurse entrepreneurs, venturing out on their own away from traditional settings.

The nurse intrapreneur, however, is a highly skilled person who creates an innovative project or program within an organized system like a hospital. In this type of enterprise, the nurse assumes complete responsibility for carrying out the effort, and usually operates out of a hospital-based clinic or office. An example might be a certified oncology nurse with his or her own cadre of patients on which assessments, histories, treatments, and post-discharge care are performed. The nurse continues to work closely with physicians who are generally the source of patient referral.

Nurse intrapreneurs may also function as a self-managed group that runs a special unit in the facility, perhaps for people with certain health problems such as asthma or emphysema. The method for paying the nurse providers will depend on their arrangement with the employing institution. Some of the options include profit-sharing, royalties, or direct payment.

The Working Climate: Patterns and Perks

Nurses of the 1990s not only have a big stake in how the working environment operates, but they play an increasingly active role in determining policies and protocols on their own units. Shared governance has empowered staff nurses to participate in decisions affecting their practice. Councils on nursing education, nursing practice, and other areas bring them together with nurse administrators to explore department-wide issues. RNs also serve on a number of hospital committees, task forces, and focus groups with members of the team including physicians, social workers, nutritionists, and other health professionals.

Employment patterns for nurses have become remarkably flexible in recent years. Self-scheduling provides a number of options, making it possible to have the best of two worlds—within and outside the hospital. Some institutions also hire per diem and part-time nurses.

On several clinical units, especially ICUs, many RNs seem to favor the 12-hour three-day shift although the traditional 8-hour five-day week still holds appeal. Since weekends tend to create staffing problems, the idea of being able to work for 24 hours and get paid for 36 can be quite intriguing. Also, the more unpopular shifts, such as evenings and nights, draw nurses seeking a 12-hour shift, a shorter week, and top pay.

There are staff nurses who favor the night shift, which in some places functions from 9:00 P.M. to 7:00 A.M. (10 hours) on a four-day schedule. They enjoy the hours because patients are awake and there is an opportunity to talk with them and their families. Also, they know that people often become more anxious at night, fearful of being alone (even with a relative present). This awareness on the part of nurses is important because they need to be available to comfort the person.

Hospital nursing offers the advantage of career mobility to RNs who want to advance upward or transfer to other practice settings. Clinical ladders, which have existed for some time, provide an opportunity for more status as well as financial reward. Usually, they consist of four or five steps or levels which indicate certain criteria to be met, such as additional education, presenting papers, publishing, research activity, and so on. Some institutions have introduced both management and clinical tracks, depending on the goals of the nurse participant.

In addition to clinical ladders, other reward systems exist. Included among these are internal promotions, nurse-of-the-month (or year) awards, perfect attendance awards, and special citations for excellence in practice. Full-time nurses, who want to continue with their formal education while working, may apply for tuition reimbursement. Some hospitals are very generous in their allocation, and may even apply their tuition policy to spouses and eligible children.

Eager to retain a competent nursing staff and reduce the possibility of fast turnover, the modern hospital offers an amazing number of perks in addition to a sound financial package covering health insurance and other benefits. It would be difficult not to be impressed with a facility that arranges for well and sick child care, elder care, subsidized housing, relocation assistance in some cases, continuing education funding, free parking, and fully equipped physical fitness centers.

*   *   *

As the primary practice site for beginning nurses, hospitals and medical centers serve as an excellent training ground for propelling them on to a successful and long-term career track. Beyond the desirable compensation and benefits package, remember that the greatest satisfaction will be derived from the nurse's ability to give nursing care of the highest quality.

This overview of nursing in a hospital reflects the complexity as well as similarities and variations in the nature, purpose, and services of these health care institutions. One fact is clear: *Nurses as the largest number of caregivers have the knowledge and skills to make a difference in the care of patients.*

The next few chapters will take you into the lives of several committed registered nurses working in various settings and with unique populations. They will share first-hand the exciting challenges they experience in everyday professional practice.

4

The Joy of Diversity:
Nurses in Action

The roles of nurses are as diverse as the settings in which they practice. As you now know, a potpourri of opportunities exist for the RN who wishes to work in a hospital or medical center. For some nurses, it might be the medical-surgical unit or emergency department, whereas others will be drawn to pediatrics, orthopaedics, or some other specialty unit. Many nurses thrive on the pace of hospital nursing where patients are discharged every day as new ones arrive on the scene. The health care team is mobilized into action, prepared to meet any or all fresh challenges.

CLINICAL NURSING:
THE INPATIENT SCENE

Critical Care Nursing

> *It was nine thirty in the evening when the ambulance rushed 55-year-old Carl Peters to Alpha Medical Center. His boss told Peters that morning that his annual evaluation was coming up in a few days. All day he had anxieties and could feel the familiar tightening in his abdomen from a chronic ulcer problem. The pounding headache didn't help either, so*

*he doctored himself with aspirins as well as the usual antacids.
Nausea and weakness soon overtook him followed by hemor-
rhaging from the mouth, and his alarmed wife called the
family physician. When informed of Peters' pending hospitalization and a tentative diagnosis of a bleeding ulcer, Frank
Davis, charge nurse on the medical intensive care unit, knew
that certain services had to be immediately available. He
alerted his staff as well as other appropriate people regarding
x-rays, blood work and other lab tests, possible transfusions,
and equipment for gastroenterology procedures. By the time
Peters reached the critical care unit, the team was waiting
and ready to begin its work.*

Intensive care units—and the specialty of critical care that
began with them—have come a long way since they were introduced in the late 1950s and early 1960s. Today, the American Association of Critical Care Nurses is the largest specialty nursing
organization in the world. Authorities in the field predict that in
time the general hospital will become one big intensive care unit.
As the number of beds begins to shrink, only the sickest patients
will be housed.

As an increasingly complex field, critical care requires expert
skills in clinical decision making. There is no other specialty in
which you can learn so much in one day. Just ask Joyce Keeler, a
17-year veteran with critical care credentials as a certified neonatal intensive care nurse (see Figure 4.1).

Keeler's home base is the UCLA Medical Center, a large teaching hospital, where she holds the title of Clinical Nurse III/Senior
Transport Nurse in the 20-bed neonatal intensive care unit
(NICU), which admits all high-risk newborns. Several RNs cover
each 12-hour shift, monitoring the infants closely. "The sickest babies need the least amount of hands-on-care," says Keeler. "They
require rest and as little handling as possible."

Family teaching begins the first day the infant comes to the
unit. "We encourage parents to visit. And although in some cases
they are not permitted to pick up the child if it is very sick, we
show them how to stroke the baby," Keeler points out. "When the

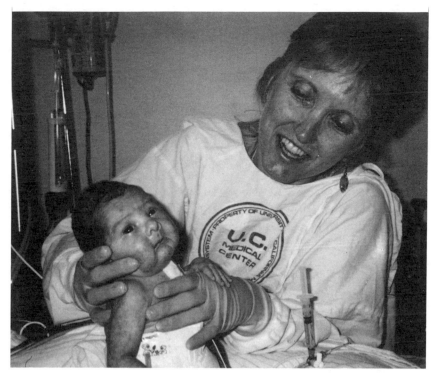

Figure 4.1 Joyce Keeler, neonatal transport nurse at UCLA Medical Center, with high-risk infant.

condition is more stable, the parents learn how to hold as well as diaper the infant properly."

As a transport nurse (flight nurse), one of the most satisfying aspects of her job is bringing critically ill infants from an outlying hospital to the medical center, caring for them, and then discharging them. She describes the NICU as a "loving unit," stressing that even children with a short life span need love. "But happily, most of our babies go home."

Keeler's reserve status with the U.S. Air Force over the past decade has paid off. She spent a three-month tour of active duty in the Persian Gulf, flying patients from Saudi Arabia to Germany. In October 1993, she was deployed for 90 days with the Air Force supporting Operation Restore Hope. "At that time I was seven weeks in Somalia in the movement of 200 patients from that country to Cairo." During that stint, Keeler participated in a number of activities that included coordinating missions with UN personnel from other nations, which "offered me a wide range of experiences."

Summing up her professional life, Keeler claims that she "still loves being a nurse." In military nursing, she states that RNs are treated and respected as officers and then as nurses. "At UCLA, we help teach the interns and residents and are recognized for our expertise."

For several years, she has participated in the annual reunion at UCLA's Medical Plaza, held for former patients in the NICU and their families. "The parents like to show off their kids, and we love to see them."

Transplant Nursing

> *Jeremy Kent had been through a lot and within a short period. Only 38-years-old, he suddenly fell ill with a severe viral infection that settled in his heart. His condition became life threatening when he developed cardiomyopathy, and the only hope of survival was a heart transplant. The thought of such surgery terrified him at first. "Will I live through the operation?" "How will I feel with someone else's heart?" "Will I ever feel normal again?" Only time would tell. After the surgery, Kent slowly opened his eyes and gazed around the unfamiliar looking room. His vision was partly blocked by curtains draped around cubicles enclosing other beds in the cardiovascular surgical intensive care unit. Becoming more oriented to the surroundings, he looked at the nurse smiling down at him and gently squeezing his hand. "How do you feel, Mr. Kent?" she asked. "I'm alive. I'm alive," he whispered happily, and drifted into a restful sleep.*

Few gifts are more precious than an organ donated to help someone else live. This generous act, in many cases a person's last act, makes it possible for adults as well as children who have heart, kidney, lung, liver, and other organ diseases to look forward to a better quality of life. Patients diagnosed with end-stage organ failure now have an 80 to 90 percent chance of surviving for one year and 70 percent for five years.

Prolonging life through high technology, such as transplantation, drugs, treatment, and mechanical devices has become an everyday occurrence. Almost every major hospital is performing some type of organ or tissue procedure. During the past ten years, the advent of transplantation has created new roles for nurses. Included is the transplant coordinator, who oversees the patient's care every step of the way, from evaluating surgical candidates through organizing their discharge and post-discharge care.

Mary Jo Modica heads the 31-bed private transplant unit at Ohio State University Medical Center in Columbus. Here, liver recipients, as well as kidney and pancreas recipients, are brought from the surgical intensive care unit (SICU). The patients range in age from 20 to 55 years and are hospitalized for 21 days.

"When admitted to us, they are very sick, weak, and sometimes confused, but in 10 to 12 days they begin to feel better. Most of them turn the corner in two weeks," reports Modica. "Many are jaundiced before the surgery, but afterwards you can almost see their color change before your eyes."

Modica's staff consists of 18 RNs, licensed practical nurses on all shifts, and certified pharmacology aides. "We prefer hiring nurses with critical care background, but we will take new graduates who can enroll in our six-month internship program if they wish to," says Modica. "Since emotional support is a large part of care, we need more nurses who understand behavior modification and change."

What Modica likes about her work is that although she does not have direct clinical responsibilities, she knows all her patients and the needs of her staff. "Helping the nurses to grow and to solve problems is very rewarding."

A nurse manager for almost four years, she formerly was a staff nurse on the SICU and on the transplant unit. Away from the working environment, she contributes her professional expertise to the International Transplant Nurses Society where she serves on the board of directors.

Also in transplant nursing for the past eight years is Thomas Steeves, a staff/charge nurse at Abbott-Northwestern Hospital in Minneapolis, Minnesota, a tertiary, teaching community institution. In October 1985, heart transplants were initiated, followed three years later by the first heart-and-lung transplantation (see Figure 4.2).

Steeves points out that after surgery the patient is brought to the cardiovascular SICU. "Here we have six-bed suites, all private rooms equipped with positive air flow and high-efficiency air to

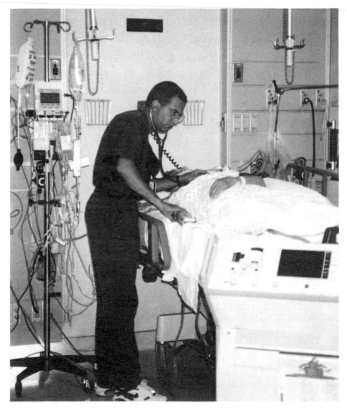

Figure 4.2 Thomas Steeves gives one-to-one nursing care to a transplant patient in the cardiovascular ICU at Abbott-Northwestern Hospital in Minneapolis.

minimize contaminants." For every transplant patient fresh from the operating room, there are two RNs assigned to at least the first shift and sometimes longer. "One nurse concentrates on bedside care—all hands on—while the other nurse takes care of lab work, medications, and physician and family contact."

When patients are ready to come off the ventilator and infusion drips and are stable, they should be ready for the telemetry unit, where the nurse and post-transplant coordinator begin discharge teaching. "Before leaving the hospital, patients must be reasonably independent and able to handle their own medicine," Steeves explains.

He characterizes his work as making a difference in people's lives. "We feel as though we are taking part in giving them a tomorrow. And many come back to see their nurses when they return for a visit."

Orthopaedic Nursing

> *During practice for an upcoming gymnastic event, 14-year-old Peggy Jean had a freak accident causing torn ligaments in her right knee. After inpatient surgery, she remained for a few days on the orthopaedic unit. Although her knee would be immobilized for six weeks, Peggy Jean was able to move around on crutches. Physical therapy would be initiated later. The teenager had one big worry while she was in the hospital—that she would never be able to continue with her gymnastic activities. By the time she was ready for discharge, however, Peggy Jean felt a lot better. The doctor and her primary nurse had both reassured her that eventually she would be "as good as new."*

Orthopaedic nursing is rapidly becoming one of the most attractive, as well as important, specialties in health care. Radical changes stemming from complex technology, advances in managing pain, and progress in research have generated new treatments and creative nursing approaches. You can be assured that the days of people suspended in traction are almost over!

Orthopaedic nurses care for patients of all ages with musculoskeletal problems caused by injuries and congenital disorders as well as by degenerative, inflammatory, metabolic, and other disorders. They practice in a variety of settings, such as special hospital units and emergency departments, trauma centers, ambulatory centers, operating rooms, post-anesthesia care units, extended care facilities, health promotion clinics, and rehabilitation centers. In some hospitals, orthopaedic units are taking on the look of a total joint replacement center.

A former orthopaedic O.R. nurse, Linda Anderson is the top RN at the Arthritis Care Center of the 750-bed Baptist Hospital in Nashville, Tennessee, home of Music City, USA, the Grand Ole Opry, and a host of recording studios. "We are one of the first comprehensive centers of this type in the nation," says Anderson who has been on board since its inception just eight years ago.

As manager of the facility, she oversees a professional staff of nurses, a counselor, and physical and occupational therapists. They provide inpatient, outpatient, and rehabilitation services. "It has been very successful working together along with the orthopaedist as a real team."

Anderson teaches classes for the patients having joint replacements. "We average 55 of these surgeries each month and the length of stay is about four or five days." She notes that preadmission workups are done prior to the operation.

One of the center's most progressive efforts is "Learning to Live," an in-house rehabilitation program created in 1988 for arthritis patients with uncontrollable pain, problems with movement, and with self-care. "The patients accepted into the program (only five at a time) have to meet certain requirements," says Anderson. "They have not responded to outpatient treatment, are medically stable, and are willing to participate in intensive educational and physical activities."

The patients arrive on Sunday and leave the following Friday. "We try to get a good fit—folks who will be compatible with one another. One of the staff's jobs is to encourage lots of interaction," explains Anderson.

The program aims to show the participants how to reduce pain, improve their ability to do daily tasks, and to move and walk. Every day, they have exercises, morning whirlpool therapy, group classes, and one-to-one evaluations. "The medication classes are important, since these patients require several drugs daily," notes Anderson. "The nurses explain the different medicines and how to take them, as well as possible side effects." Family members are welcome to attend the classes and activities.

The nurses do a great deal of teaching in the program. "In the cooking classes, we show the patients how to use certain equipment like built up utensils," says Anderson. At discharge, each participant receives a calendar containing a list of daily tasks to continue at home, such as paraffin baths, or wearing splints to lessen or prevent deformities.

Two and four weeks later, the center's nurses contact the people to check on their progress and invite them to return in two months to be checked. "Many patients have become good friends in the meantime, as well as one another's support group," states Anderson. "They tell us that the week spent here in 'Learning to Live' has changed their lives."

Maternity Nursing—Nurse-Midwifery

> *"Here's your new daughter, Mrs. Carroll," said Alicia Kane, gently placing the infant on her mother's abdomen. "It's what we call bonding," added the certified nurse-midwife who had delivered the child a few minutes earlier. For Tim and Kathy Carroll, it was the supreme joy of their life with the birth of Baby Beth. Kathy had enjoyed her pregnancy and particularly liked the care and attention given to her by Nurse Kane. "You always have time to listen to both Tim and me and answer all our questions," she said. "And we appreciate that very much."*

Historically, nursing has played a crucial role in advancing women's health. In the 20th century, maternal and child care has come far from the days when women in labor were physically restrained, heavily draped, and numbed with anesthesia. The evolution of the modern nurse-midwife has been a significant development in the nursing profession and is a highly satisfying career for RNs pursuing this specialty.

Not all nurses, however, who are involved in obstetric and neonatal nursing follow the path of nurse midwifery. Many staff nurses assist physicians and certified nurse-midwives (CNMs) during and following the birth, with some working in the hospital nursery and others attending to the care of the mother on the unit. Patient turnover is generally fast, with discharges within 24 to 48 hours barring complications.

In the United States, some 6,000 certified nurse-midwives are working in birthing centers, hospital maternity units, perinatal clinics, and other settings. According to the American College of Nurse-Midwives, the certifying body for CNMs, the practice of midwifery includes services to healthy women and their babies, such as prenatal care, labor and delivery management, postpartum care, well women gynecology, and normal newborn care. Between 1975 and 1991, the number of hospital births attended by CNMs jumped nearly seven-fold from almost 20,000 to more than 158,000.

"One of the interesting aspects of our practice is the preconception class we offer to families who consider having a child," says Jan Kriebs, a CNM employed by the Johns Hopkins University School of Medicine in Baltimore. Less than a year in her present position, she worked previously for a health maintenance organization where she did prenatal and postpartum care and family planning for the HMO employees. During that period, she delivered all her maternity patients at a Washington, DC hospital.

At Hopkins, she shares a practice with Carolyn Gegor and another CNM. They are employed by the university, providing care at the hospital to both the privately insured and medical assistance patients. "Because we are an academic practice, we are also involved in ongoing research and formal teaching," Kriebs reports.

The patients have the option of delivering their babies in birth rooms or in the traditional labor delivery suite in the hospital. The nurse-midwife's responsibilities, however, begin much earlier. "All three of us get to know our patients well before their babies are born," says Kriebs.

She points out that the CNM must be willing and able to develop a management plan covering every aspect of her patient's care. "We look at not only the immediate and short-term needs but also a long-range plan. You have to integrate today's care into a lifetime of health."

In their practice, the CNMs spend a lot of time with their patients, sharing information and listening to their concerns. "During the first visit, I do a complete health, nutritional, and social history along with a physical examination. Many of the clinic patients are high risk, including drug abusers who have premature labor and low-birthweight babies," says Kriebs.

As clinical director of the Fetal Assessment Center, Gegor works closely with the staff nurses there. She also teaches sonograph skills to the perinatal nurses, nurse-midwives, and obstetrical residents. "What offers me a long time reward in nursing is the continuity of caring for women during their pregnancy as well as caring for their well woman GYN and family planning needs," she declares.

Her colleague Jan Kriebs refers to herself as a "career changer" since she already had a BA degree in another field (speech and theater), and was the mother of a toddler when she decided to become a nurse. "I was seeking a profession that would enable me to work with women's health issues. Nursing offered an accessible route to begin practice so that I could finance enough education to do what I really wanted—to work directly with women as a health care provider."

Kriebs eventually earned a master's degree in nursing and her credential as a certified nurse-midwife. One thing she is sure of: "This is what I wanted and this is where I intend to stay!"

Hyperbaric Nursing

"He's got the Bends!" That's how Gary Brown described his co-worker Marsh Philips. Both men worked as deep sea divers, but the last time they went down, Philips came up too rapidly. He suffered great pain which caused uncontrollable bodily

contortions. Brown and some of the crew rushed their friend to the hospital and treatment immediately followed. The patient was placed in a hyperbaric chamber so that the air pressure could return at a level to which he was originally exposed.

While undergoing this kind of therapy, whether used for the Bends (otherwise known as "decompression sickness") or some other condition, the affected person will require the skillful intervention of the hyperbaric nurse. In the heart of Middle America at the University of Kansas Medical Center in Kansas City, Ruth Rampey-Dobbs and Linda Appleton jointly staff a two-chamber hyperbaric unit. Recently, Louis Nicholson was employed to give technical assistance.

Recruited when the new unit opened in January 1994, both RNs had worked previously with Nicholson in the hospital's 10-bed burn center, which housed critically ill patients with thermal injuries. "The burn center required a special type of nurse, who must have understanding plus excellent medical-surgical skills," says Rampey-Dobbs. "But in my present job, the biggest need is for the emotional care of the patients."

She and Appleton point out that the idea of being enclosed in a large, cylindrical chamber can be quite frightening, even if it is only for 90 minutes. "So, what we do initially is give patients the necessary information and urge them to ask questions." The most important thing, they add, is to establish trust from the very beginning.

Patients are admitted to the hyperbaric unit for a number of reasons, the most common being for wounds that don't heal, carbon monoxide poisoning, and skin grafts that won't take as quickly as they should. Once confined to the chamber, the person receives pure compressed oxygen, which increases oxygen in the blood and tissues. "The nurses have to monitor the patient's vital signs very carefully so as to avert any complications," explains Rampey-Dobbs.

Inside the compact, stationary chamber, the person is able to turn, watch television hooked up on the outside, and communicate easily with the staff, who can be seen and heard clearly through their microphone. Families are encouraged to remain on the unit with their loved one.

Following the treatment, the nurse dresses the patient's wounds if indicated. Discharge can be to home or to the appropriate unit in the hospital. In cases of chronic wounds, treatment often continues on a daily basis for about three weeks.

The nurses' schedule may involve the care of seven or eight patients a day. Every other week, Rampey-Dobbs and Appleton alternate being on call after the usual working hours. "And we do get called," exclaims Rampey-Dobbs. "We go to the emergency room and screen the patient for possible admission to the hyperbaric unit."

She notes that the results of the treatment have been wonderful. "And we always let our patients know that *they* are the boss!"

AMBULATORY NURSING:
THE OUTPATIENT SCENE

For decades, nurses have provided care to patients in a variety of clinics located in the outpatient departments of hospitals. The structure and operation of these clinics, however, have undergone marked change in recent times. At present, a number of outpatient facilities house large specialized centers, offering services to patients with particular health problems.

Many cancer centers, for example, have day treatment units where patients come for chemotherapy, radiation therapy, hydration, special antibiotics, and other medications. Headed and staffed by nurses certified in oncology nursing, these ambulatory centers can treat as many as 90 patients a day. The nurses coordinate the plan of care with other health care workers, and arrange support groups according to the person's diagnosis.

What has taken on a new look in the past ten years is the face of same day surgery, performed on people of all ages. Once the exclusive purview of the inpatient operating room, an impressive number of surgeries have been shifted to the outpatient setting. Among this group are hernia repairs, breast biopsies, orthopaedic hand operations, and a host of other procedures.

In many places, ambulatory nurses assume responsibility for educating and preparing patients in advance of their operations.

They schedule them to meet with the staff nurse who does a head-to-toe assessment. In a teaching room, patients often can look at videotapes related to their upcoming surgery.

For children undergoing tonsillectomies and procedures involving pressure-equalizing tubes for ear problems, some hospitals book a certain day as Children's Day. The youngsters have picture books that are distributed to the offices of their physician. The visuals may even show the layout of the day surgery unit along with stories written at the child's level. Following the operation, young patients may receive a teddy bear dressed in O.R. greens or blues.

As day surgery and other clinic services continue to expand, a whole set of fresh challenges awaits the nurse who chooses to work in ambulatory care. On the rise are procedures that require different skills and more advanced technology. Newer outpatient surgery, such as cholecystectomy (removal of a gall bladder), or lithotripsy (crushing of kidney stones), may appear still dramatic but in time will become more commonplace.

Day Surgery

At Seattle's Virginia Mason Medical Center, over 6,000 lithotripsies have been performed since May 1985. "We are now considered the stone center of a wide area," claims staff nurse, Joanna Boatman. Along with two part-time RNs, she is assigned exclusively to this area in the hospital's short-stay services department.

"We begin at seven and work until we get done," she says, noting that their workload consists of scheduling about ten patients per week. After the procedure, the patient is taken to the recovery room for a couple of hours. "Most people return home the same day, but some will remain overnight if the surgery is done in the early evening."

Two weeks later, the nurses mail a questionnaire to patients to determine any problems and to find out if they have contacted their physician. In three months, another survey is sent for additional information. Complications are rare with lithotripsy.

Boatman, who also has another commitment as president of Washington Women United, a political organization devoted to women's issues, likes the autonomy of her job and "being able to predict what's next."

Specialized Services

Throughout our nation's health care communities, nurses are valiantly contributing to the care and comfort of persons infected with the HIV virus. Nurses are helping patients and their loved ones to cope by providing intense education to extend life and sustain its quality as long as possible.

Working in the special immunology service of Children's National Medical Center in Washington, DC, two professional nurses, Catherine Ernsthausen and Kimberly Bright, are devoted to the care of HIV-infected youngsters. Ernsthausen, a pediatric nurse practitioner with a master's degree from University of Rochester (NY), came on board in August 1994. A veteran of nine years at the hospital, Bright holds a baccalaureate from Howard University. Their work involves early detection of HIV in children of infected mothers, and the treatment of youngsters already diagnosed as HIV positive.

Ernsthausen points out that HIV-infected women transmit the virus to their infants 20 to 30 percent of the time. "The challenge is to determine which children are infected with HIV soon after birth so that treatment can begin as soon as possible. All babies should be evaluated, starting as early as four weeks."

She further notes the reluctance of parents to have their baby seen because they fear it might have the HIV virus. "Much education and support are offered by the entire special immunology team at each step of the diagnosis and treatment."

Based in the outpatient clinic, the nurses see approximately 40 to 50 patients each week. Ernsthausen notes that with new patients, she elicits from the parent the family medical history. She also assesses the child's progress, looking for indicators of HIV infection. When the laboratory results are ready from the first interview, she shares them in person with the mother or father.

"Patient education begins at the first visit," says Bright, who does histories, assessments, weighing and measuring the children, and administering medications. "I'm really close to the families whom I see over a long period of time. And I like the age group."

Pastoral counseling as well as support groups conducted by social workers are available. Also on the staff are two research nurse-coordinators who monitor the patients on active protocols, two physicians, a psychologist, nutritionist, and administrative personnel. "The team is following about 150 HIV-positive children between the ages of birth and twelve-years-old, in addition to those whose HIV status has yet to be determined," says Ernsthausen.

She characterizes her young patients as the real heroes. "They are showing me how to live in the midst of overwhelming illness and sometimes depressing social conditions. And the opportunity to help families work toward optimal health in a caring and compassionate way is what makes my job so satisfying."

Comprehensive Services: Modular Approach

San Francisco's Veterans Administration Medical Center, which operates one of the most progressive ambulatory care centers on the West Coast, initiated modular groupings of several clinics in 1989. "We reorganized primarily to offer better continuity of care to patients," says Sherry Koski, associate chief of nursing service for ambulatory care. "Also, by having the same charge nurse consistently in the module, communication and morale have improved greatly among nurses, physicians, and the clerks."

Matrix management was introduced before the modules. "Each week, representatives of nursing, medicine, medical administration, social services, pharmacy, and lab meet to coordinate our ambulatory activities and do some problem solving," Koski adds.

How does the nursing staff feel about the modular approach? Tess Beltran, a twenty-two-year professional in the VA system can tell you. She and other charge nurses in their respective modules treat patients in a variety of assigned clinics, such as GI, urology, oncology, and STAMP—a special team for amputations, mobility, prosthetics/orthotics, arrhythmia, chest, heart-thoracic, liver disease, and arthritis. "We now have more patient and staff satisfaction as well as improved efficiency," declares Beltran, who works from Monday through Friday.

On the average, she interacts with about 30 patients a day (all veterans). Besides patient teaching, she also coordinates the person's care with the hospital's home care service and consults with visiting nurses. "The patients know they can call me whenever they like."

Each module has established an RN follow-up clinic. "Our goal is to provide a way for scheduling a patient's appointment with the nurse for close monitoring and education. It's a new link in discharge planning," says Beltran. Patients come to the RN follow-up clinic for injections, dressings, blood pressure check, and an assessment of their general condition. They do not usually see the physician at that time.

Another facet of Beltran's work is becoming involved in the patient's support system. "We are concerned with the person as a whole, and that includes the family. It is so rewarding, particularly when they come back and say 'Thank you. You've helped us a lot.'"

* * *

Sharing these real life experiences has probably given you a better idea of some of the hospital specialties and settings that attract nurses. Keep in mind, however, that RNs also perform their clinical skills in dialysis units, operating rooms, emergency departments, and several other areas.

Working in a hospital represents an exciting arena for many nurses who wouldn't have it any other way. What emerges is a fascinating contrast between the mystical and the very real. Drama appears to be the daily watchword, with health professionals playing various roles while their patients take center stage. You can be certain that life will never be dull for RNs who set their sights on a big medical center or a smaller community hospital. The action will always be there!

5

The Community: New Frontiers for Nurses

Although the majority of nurses are employed by hospitals at the present time, the shift to the community is already underway and expected to intensify in the coming decade. Fifteen percent (250,000) of RNs now work in state or local health departments, nonhospital-based home health agencies, various types of community centers, student services, and occupational health.

You're undoubtedly familiar with the term *public health nursing* which is often used interchangeably with *community health nursing*. Public health nurses (PHNs) focus on such activities as health promotion and disease prevention, community health protection, and assistance to gaining access to care. They practice in agencies carrying the title of public health, home health, community health, or visiting nurse.

Some public health nurses work in schools, outpatient clinics, community health centers, free walk-in clinics for drug addiction and sexually transmitted diseases, migrant labor camps, and rural areas. Others are employed by hospitals that conduct home care programs, or serve as a link between the facility and the community.

One of the unique aspects of public health nursing is the autonomy or freedom afforded the nurse. You are on your own in a setting "without walls," which requires knowledge and good clinical judgment as well as the ability to adapt to many types of environments. You can expect to provide services to people of different ethnic, cultural, and socioeconomic backgrounds, living in neighborhoods that may range from well-to-do high-rise apartments to shelters for the less fortunate.

At some point in your career as a public health nurse, you may wish to broaden your vistas and seek new experiences and new sites. A worthwhile move could be signing up with the government's Indian Health Service, and joining other colleagues working on reservations in some of the nation's western communities. There, nurses give direct care along with health teaching and maintenance. Because of the high incidence of diabetes in the Indian population, some RNs seek advanced preparation and become certified as diabetes educators.

Home Health Nursing

Public health nurses find considerable satisfaction working in home care agencies, such as Visiting Nurse Associations. "Healing at Home" is how the Visiting Nurse Service of New York characterizes its mission. This legendary organization, which evolved from the vision of Lillian Wald and her Henry Street nurses over 100 years ago, continues its home care tradition.

As a key component of the nation's changing health care system, home health programs provide for teams of health workers to give medical and skilled nursing care and supervision, personal day care, housekeeping and dietary services, social day care, social transportation, and home improvement and maintenance. Often described as nursing at its finest, home care makes it clinically safe for hospital patients to be discharged earlier, whether it's a person convalescing from a hip joint replacement, a new mother who had a Caesarean delivery, or a young adult with AIDS on antibiotic infusions.

What Margaret Moran finds most satisfying about her job as a home health staff nurse is working with a variety of patients and families and making independent decisions. For almost 12 years, she has been in practice for the Visiting Nurse Association of Eastern Montgomery County in Willow Grove, Pennsylvania, and continues to find her job stimulating.

The agency, the home care department of Abington Memorial Hospital, employs 100 RNs, of whom 50 percent are part-time or relief status. Supervised by the nurses, certified home health aides working for the agency, or those available through contracts, assist patients with personal care and related services.

Moran's "beat" covers part of Horsham Township where she sees on the average six patients a day and spends about a half hour with each one. She also has responsibilities at the agency's headquarters, completing required documentation and having conferences with other health professionals involved in the patient's care, such as physical, occupational, or speech therapists, and medical social workers.

In the field, she gives hands-on care, assessment and instruction in such areas as diabetic management, wound care, management of tube feedings, chemo and radiation therapy follow-up, and evaluation of heart patients.

"Much of my job consists of teaching patients and their families how to manage their care. For example, how to handle needle equipment, diet information, medications—including those given intravenously—and home safety," explains Moran. "Our goal is to make the patient and the family as independent as possible."

Her caseload consists of an adult population, with a large number requiring geriatric care. The more common health problems are diabetes, heart and vascular conditions, cancer, and pulmonary disease. "On a first visit to a new patient, I do a health history and physical assessment to determine the patient's problems and needs," says Moran. "I also arrange for blood work, clarify the person's medications, and follow through with the physician on any abnormal findings."

She likes the schedule arranged by the agency. With two teenage children, the hours are convenient. "It's not always easy to work full time while raising a family, but it can be done." How does she manage it? "Set limits and put some things on the back burner," she declares. "And a supportive husband always helps!"

Nursing: The Career of a Lifetime

School Health/College Health

Approximately 26,000 professional nurses work in public and private schools throughout the nation, where they deliver primary health care to children and youth. They should all be clinically prepared to work with students of every age and special needs.

Think back to your own childhood and perhaps an experience with the school nurse, and it may remind you of a person whose main job was to soothe a child with a minor fall or apply a Band-Aid® to a small abrasion or cut on the knee. That may have been the case at one time, probably eons ago, but the school nurse's ancient trademark of only *First Aid* has happily been supplemented by programs involving health teaching, environmental health, and safety. The scope of these activities, however, as well as how they will be implemented, depends to some extent on the wishes of the community and the actions of the school council or board.

Although some school districts employ their own nurses, others contract with a local public health agency. School nurses work with other school health personnel in fostering national education goals. They must ensure that children come to school ready to learn, and that problems involving substance abuse and related concerns be addressed.

In addition to liking young people and meeting their health needs, school nurses find the convenience of their work schedule a big plus in their job. One of the newer trends in the field is the introduction of school-based or school-linked clinics, in which school nurse practitioners provide a wide range of services. Over 150 of these school health centers have evolved, with a growing number already on the horizon.

Many nurses opt to practice in college or university health programs because of the stimulating environment. Most college health services operate on an ambulatory basis although some have small infirmaries. The activities are geared mainly to the students, who pay a health fee entitling them to certain benefits. Faculty and campus employees may also use the service as needed.

A certified college health nurse, Elizabeth Bosselman joined the Columbia University Health Service on a temporary basis in

1986. She liked it so much that a year later she decided to stay on. "It was my best professional move," she says. A former school nurse in her hometown of Gloucester, Massachusetts, Bosselman has enjoyed working with both the younger children and the college-age population.

"But there is a difference in job expectations with the two groups. In the public school system, you cannot treat a child without the parent's permission—not even to have an X-ray taken," she explains. "With college students, you view them as really emancipated. They have developed their own uniqueness and like to experiment with different life-styles."

Located on the second floor of one of the campus buildings, the Health Service employs seven ambulatory staff nurses, ten nurse practitioners, and seven physicians representing various specialties. The facility houses nine examining rooms where the staff see approximately 300 patients each day, including those treated in the Women's Health Center on the fourth floor.

Like the other RNs, Bosselman's responsibilities are as diversified as the kinds of health problems and needs she must deal with continually. "In one day I may start off early in the morning giving allergy shots and other injections," she states. "There is a lot of overseas travel among the students and faculty who require vaccinations. It could be an anthropology major who plans to spend a year in some exotic place like the rain forest in Brazil, or a business student eager to explore potential opportunities in one of Africa's developing nations."

Bosselman also works in the triage booth screening patients who have different complaints, with the more common being ear infections that require irrigations, sprained ankles, and injuries from contact sports. "We do testing for HIV infection at the request of the student. An HIV clinic is available in the evening for those testing positive. All information about students is kept confidential and not reported to their family."

She observes that at this youthful stage of their lives, the students can experience a host of problems. Some come to the Health Service depressed and anxious, stressed out from studying. Eating disorders are not uncommon in this age group. "And there's too much cigarette smoking," she asserts.

"The nurses try to get as much information as possible while listening carefully. We usually refer the patient first to a physician for a complete checkup and then follow through if indicated." There are also group classes and special counseling.

Health education is a large part of the program at the Health Service. Bosselman notes that volunteer students are trained to go into the dormitories once a week as peer health counselors. "They discuss safe sex and related concerns, presenting their message in a creative skit format called the 'Dr. Whoopee show.' And it goes over in a big way!"

How does she feel about her career in college health? "I love it," she responds enthusiastically. "I enjoy talking with the students, and, of course, learning from them."

The Community Nursing Center/Primary Health Care

Some people say that community nursing centers are the best kept secret in American health care. Since the mid-1980s, they have begun to spring up across the country. More than half are affiliated with a facility, such as a home health agency, retirement community, or public health department. Many are linked to university schools of nursing while others are freestanding.

One of the most attractive features of community nursing centers is that the nurse occupies a chief management position. RNs control their own practice and are accountable and responsible for the care of their patients. As an alternative model in rural health delivery, they offer access to care and comprehensive services.

Ever since it opened in April 1994, the Tri-County Community Health Center has had a booming "business," in serving the health needs of the residents in the northwestern part of Illinois. "We have had over 2000 visits," says Bette Chilton, the director and a certified specialist in community health, who joined the Center from the outset as a primary developer in the project. She describes the building, which is located on the campus of Kishwaukee College in Malta, as literally being in the middle of one big cornfield!

Operating on a five-year grant to Northern Illinois University from the Division of Nursing, U.S. Public Health Service, the project has been a dream come true for the medically underserved, underinsured people in Dekalb, Ogle, and Lee Counties.

"This is the first community health center to provide affordable primary health care in the area," Chilton points out. "Many of the patients are the working poor and qualify for a 50 percent fee reduction."

Other key people working with her are four master's prepared family nurse practitioners including Mary Uscian, former Center director who holds an academic appointment at Northern Illinois University. Nursing students come to the clinic as a learning site for primary care.

Clinic hours run from 8 A.M. to 4:30 P.M., Monday, Wednesday, and Friday, and 12:30 P.M. to 8 P.M. in the evening on Tuesdays and Thursdays. Staffing includes both baccalaureate and associate degree nurses. Patients consist mainly of young women and children. Chilton reports that the Center has had no known cases of HIV infection or AIDS. "Although we do screening for pregnancy, we do not take care of maternity patients. Family planning, however, is one of the services we offer."

Patient referrals come from a variety of sources. "Many have heard of us by word-of-mouth, whereas others are referred by physicians and nurses in health departments," she states. "The school nurses have been wonderful in this regard. They really have been advocates for the Center."

Among the nurses' activities are visits to shelters for homeless and abused women, the county jail, and schools where physicals are performed on the children. "In 1994, the schools had 100 percent compliance from the parents for examinations and immunizations," notes Chilton. "In the near future, we hope to provide services to day-care centers."

Every other Friday one of the FNPs confers with a physician who comes to the clinic to review patient charts and discuss any concerns. "The doctor is available at any time for consultation if I need her," Chilton explains. "Otherwise the health care is almost entirely managed by the nurses who do assessments, prescribe medications, and oversee the care plan."

Chilton is still surprised by how much has been accomplished within a relatively short period. "It is thrilling to be part of what we are doing. The patients tell us that they love the service and being listened to as well as participating in their care." She adds that by showing nursing students what nurses do is "helping to educate them to be primary care providers for tomorrow."

*   *   *

In addition to the settings already described, some RNs become office nurses while others join up with large firms or institutions requiring occupational health nurses (OHNs) on the premises. As an OHN, you could aspire to be one of the lucky nurses working at the United Nations, or on the health services staff of a leading national corporation. Or how about connecting with your town's biggest department store?

Without question, compelling challenges await the nurse who enters the world of community nursing. So, set your sights, pick your spot, and go for it!

6

Nursing with
Special Populations

As you know by now, part of nursing's greatest appeal lies in the range of options open to RNs. For the moment, however, stay tuned in to learn more about nurses in clinical practice. As you read on, you may reflect on what *your* preference might be once you join the ranks of professional nursing. Will there be a particular age group that you favor over others? How about the setting—in or out of the hospital? Will you be drawn to taking care of people with particular health problems associated with surgical, pediatric, psychiatric, or neuro conditions? Whatever you decide, you can be sure of one thing: *You'll always have choices.*

The nurses sharing the following stories have also made choices in bringing their expertise to special populations. You will find their contributions heartwarming because they are dealing with important concerns affecting contemporary American life.

CONTEMPORARY CONCERNS

Geriatric Nursing

Advances in medical science as well as knowledge about healthier life-styles have made it possible for people to live longer and continue to lead productive lives. As you look around your own community, you're probably aware of the growing number of older folks. Many of them seem quite spry and active and can be characterized as the "well elderly."

Perhaps your grandmother or great aunt, or even a neighbor fit into this category. Although you can't expect to find them on the ski slopes at Stowe or Aspen (well, maybe one or two rare adventurers!), they dance, play cards, attend seminars, travel, and participate in a variety of other activities. Some older people still manage to maintain their own homes while others prefer to live in senior residential centers that provide important services including health care.

Among the elderly, however, is a large contingent with chronic diseases or conditions that require long-term care. Many have no other option than to be cared for in a nursing home, a facility structured like a hospital in some ways but functioning at a different pace.

The nursing home is a setting that offers a real challenge for the nurse as the patient's advocate. While some of the residents can move about freely and adjust to the ambience of the institution, others are relatively helpless without friends or family.

There appears to be a trend in the growing number of RNs working in nursing homes although, at present, most of the caregivers are licensed practical nurses and aides. Becoming more visible are geriatric nurse practitioners (GNPs) whose expert nursing skills have contributed markedly to improving the quality of care in these facilities. GNPs not only assess the patients (usually called "residents") and their progress, but also perform some diagnostic procedures. In addition, they explore family and personal relationships as well as related matters affecting the resident's health condition.

Geriatric nurse practitioners also work in other settings. Take Chris Davitt, for example, a master's prepared RN, who earned her ANA certification in 1994. For the past six years, she has practiced in the Center for Geriatric Health Care, an outpatient service of Newark-Beth Israel Medical Center in New Jersey.

On staff at the Center are two other GNPs, four attending physicians—all fellowship-trained geriatricians—four social workers, a medical technician, and support staff. Davitt reports that she usually begins her working day at 8 A.M., when she spends about an hour making rounds in the hospital checking on the geriatric patients.

"I assess their condition and consult with the nurses on the unit," she says. In addition, she does discharge planning with the social worker, which includes the possibility of nursing home placement.

For the remainder of the day, Davitt is based in the outpatient area where she sees patients with a physician, consults on pain management, and provides information and instruction on various aspects of care. Health teaching often includes family members. Her caseload consists of people over age 65, with a large number 85 years and older. She characterizes this latter group as the fastest growing population. "Our oldest woman is 102!"

Davitt points out that as people age, their health problems increase. "Our goal is to keep our population functional, healthy, and living in the community as long as possible." As part of her practice, she has a wellness program that involves visits to the elderly housed in buildings for senior citizens.

She is enthusiastic about a new project underway with the Newark Housing Authority, designed to provide health care services to approximately 15,000 elderly residents living in twelve buildings. "We are still in the early stage of determining needs," states Davitt, coordinator of the effort. "The intent is to have a health team available in each building a half a day a week."

One of the many facets of her job is serving as a preceptor to graduate nursing students from a local college, who can observe firsthand the practice of a GNP in an ambulatory setting. "I find it stimulating to teach and work with them," she notes. Another activity that she participates in each year is the health fair for senior citizens where health screenings are done, literature disseminated, and resources in the community highlighted. "We also do blood pressures, and last year we did 125 in one day!"

Davitt claims that the collaborative relationship she has with physicians and other colleagues has been extremely fulfilling. "As for the patients, they tell me how happy they are with the care," she says. "I really like older people. Each person is unique and interesting."

Addictions Nursing

Since the 1960s, the number of Americans with an addiction to drugs has been increasing yearly. The use and abuse of substances cuts across all ages and socioeconomic groups. It is believed that nearly 25 percent of all admissions to hospitals have a primary or secondary diagnosis of chemical dependency.

Accurate statistics, however, on the extent of substance abuse in the general population are difficult to pinpoint, since reporting the problem depends upon the affected person's recognition that one exists. One fact that can be supported is that 5 to 33 percent of known cases of HIV infection nationwide stem from intravenous use. In high-risk areas such as the northeast, it can range from 55 to 60 percent.

Over the last ten years, addictions nursing has come into its own as an important new specialty in the profession. According to Marion Conti-O'Hare, a nursing care coordinator at the Department of Veterans Affairs in New York City, an addicted client is a person who has lost control over a substance or any other behavior that causes difficulty in his or her life. "Disorders can range from chemical dependency to eating problems—such as anorexia or bulimia, gambling, and other types of compulsions," says Conti-O'Hare.

A clinical specialist in psychiatric and mental health nursing, she also is a certified addictions nurse and credentialled alcoholism counselor. Her practice at present lies in the area of chemical dependency, which involves addictions to substances such as alcohol, heroin, and cocaine. Since 1990, she has headed the VA hospital's four-week inpatient substance abuse and rehabilitation program, supported by a staff of RNs and nonprofessional personnel. Treatment is provided in the 22-bed detoxification unit and a 28-bed rehab unit.

Like most psychiatric health professionals, Conti-O'Hare refers to patients as clients. "We believe that the person is coming for services and therefore has a responsibility to do some things for himself in treatment. He is not coming to be dependent," she emphasizes. "Clients need to be taught to take charge of their lives to gain sobriety."

Her clients at the facility consist mostly of male veterans ranging in age from 30 to 50. "Chemical dependency can be just as common in women, but it is often hidden," she claims. "The stigma seems to be greater and the family protects them, thus making recovery more difficult."

Seventy percent of the clients represent a homeless, indigent population, and 30 to 40 percent have psychiatric or personality problems. "If their behavior becomes serious or violent, we transfer them to the psychiatric unit," reports Conti-O'Hare. "We also house people on our unit who have AIDS or are HIV positive, and many of them have additional problems, such as diabetes and tuberculosis."

On the detoxification unit, the program aims to initiate the client into recovery. Treatment consists of drug therapy, which prevents complications of withdrawal. "Through a multidisciplinary approach, we give lectures, group exercises, one-to-one counseling, and group therapy. When detox is completed, we urge clients to go directly to the rehab unit to continue the recovery process," says Conti-O'Hare.

She admits, however, that it doesn't always work out that way since 30 percent of the clients leave against medical advice. "The recidivism rate is high because the problem is not the substance but rather that people have not learned coping skills, and use drugs and alcohol to compensate for them and then become addicted."

Conti-O'Hare also points out that relapse is part of recovery and that people don't get better spontaneously. "As relapses become less frequent, the recovery is longer." During the inpatient treatment, meetings take place featuring such groups as Alcoholics Anonymous, Narcotics Anonymous, and Cocaine Anonymous.

As for her relationship with the nursing staff, Conti-O'Hare considers it important to listen and to stress how to be positive as well as nonjudgmental. "I try to be a role model." The field of addictions nursing, she believes, requires special skills and a lot of understanding. "It is hard work. But I wouldn't have it any other way."

Hospice Nursing

While the past forty years have seen cancer cure rates rise by 50 percent, the incidence rates are also higher. This means that oncology nursing remains an important field with many nurses taking up the gauntlet. According to the Oncology Nursing Society, more than three-fourths of its members are employed full time in cancer care. The majority work in hospitals at present, whereas the rest practice in ambulatory clinics, cancer centers, physicians' offices, and home care.

A hospice-oncology liaison nurse in the Cancer Center of Presbyterian Hospital in Charlotte, North Carolina, Kristine Hunt has worked since 1989 in the five-bed hospice. Adjacent to an oncology unit, the hospice has private quarters for family members, a small kitchen, and a conference room. It is staffed by a charge nurse during the day, an evening and night nurse, and a nursing assistant day and evening. "Some of the patients walk around and visit with the others," says Hunt, who is certified in both oncology nursing and hospice nursing (see Figure 6.1).

"The concept of hospice is more of a philosophy than a place. This means that families can be assisted in the care of a terminally ill patient," she explains, adding that emotional support begins with the entrance interview before the patient is admitted to the hospice. "At that time, I talk about our philosophy along with some of the physiology of the disease, lab values, and other information, such as discharge plans regarding the patient's preference. The average length of stay is 10 to 14 days."

In counseling patients and their loved ones, she helps them to understand the effects of dealing with a terminal disease, and to identify their coping mechanisms. "I do a lot of teaching about the wonderful messages a dying person gives us. Many positive interactions and resolutions can transpire if there is a guide open to all possibilities during this last journey."

One of Hunt's roles is to assess the eligibility of oncology patients in the hospital for transfer to the hospice. First, there must be assurance that there will be a primary caregiver present when the patient goes home, as many prefer to spend their last weeks in familiar surroundings. "Another criterion is that the person has

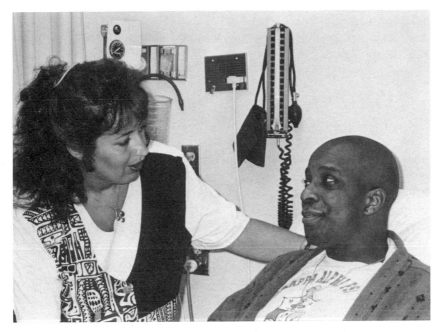

Figure 6.1 A terminally ill patient discusses end of life concerns with hospice nurse, Kristine Hunt, at Presbyterian Hospital in Charlotte, NC.

decided not to seek further curative measures," she points out. "Some continue with chemo or radiation therapy for palliative reasons, and we do give morphine for managing pain."

Much of her time is spent in case management, in which she looks at the needs for a safe discharge. "I believe in doing whatever it takes to empower a patient and family members to take control of their destiny as much as they can," she asserts. "Dealing with these patients forces you to examine your own issues regarding the fragility of life and what we take and give in this world. For all the precious moments I have shared with my patients, I will be forever grateful."

With that kind of commitment, it is no wonder that North Carolina honored Kristine Hunt in October 1994 with the "Great 100 Award." Out of more than 60,000 RNs across the state, she was one of a hundred cited for her "advanced interpersonal skills and level of professionalism demonstrating excellent oncology nursing practice."

Family Health Nursing

Some startling findings about major social and health issues, such as adolescent sexuality and pregnancy, have paved the way for new and broader roles for professional nurses. You might be interested to know that in the past five years, teenage pregnancy and birthrates in the United States have exceeded those in most developed nations. Sixty-five percent of those births are out of wedlock. Compounding the problem is the high use of hard drugs among young people, with 375,000 babies born annually to mothers using crack.

Working in Family Planning Services (FPS) in the heart of Appalachia, Dyan Aretakis brings health practices and education to an adolescent population (see Figure 6.2). The FPS program, which she launched in 1989 as project director, operates out of the OB/GYN outpatient area of the University of Virginia Health Science Center in Charlottesville. Here in rural America, in the foothills of the Blue Ridge Mountains, considerable poverty exists.

Aretakis, who is certified as both a family nurse practitioner and pediatric nurse practitioner, introduced the program by speaking to groups at community centers, housing projects, schools, and other sites. "I participated in some of the first training sessions to prepare teachers in family life education," she recalls. "Our services are much broader than just giving birth control information. The focus is on sexuality and reproductive health issues."

In her practice, she sees from 80 to 100 patients each month, ranging from 11 to 44 years of age. During the patient's first visit, she does a health history and physical assessment. If there are any problems or abnormalities, a backup physician is always available. "The health history is important. I look for signs of sexual abuse. An alarming number of patients share with me for the first time their experience with incest."

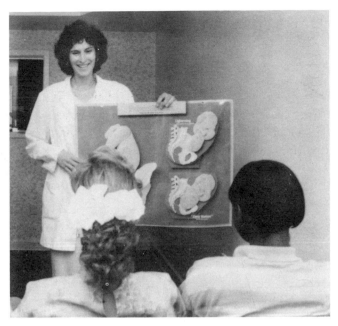

Figure 6.2 Dyan Aretakis explains infant growth and development to pregnant teenagers in her Appalachian clinic.

The repeated pregnancies of teenage girls coming to the FPS clinic led Aretakis to establish the Young Mothers Program. "We needed to educate and support pregnant adolescents. An RN conducts weekly classes and follows up on deliveries," she says.

The success of the Young Mothers Program has spurred the development of a separate outpatient facility, the Teen Health Center. "One criterion for staffing includes nurses who have good rapport with adolescents and knowledge of sexuality," reports Aretakis. "Our services include counseling and education on prenatal care, reproductive issues, and prevention of AIDS and other sexually transmitted diseases. We also bring in young men because they need information on health care."

Married and the mother of a youngster just past a year old, she admits to working long hours. "But I earn a great salary, and most of all find a lot of satisfaction in seeing the pattern of growth in what we're doing. In particular, I enjoy working with young people at a critical time in their lives."

*   *   *

The way nurses practice, in caring *about* as well as caring *for* their patients or clients, is reflected in the words they speak and the actions they take. Working with certain populations requires a special kind of person to care for people with special needs. Whatever the age, whatever the health problem, reach out and a nurse will be there.

7

The Educational Program: Finding the Right Fit

Nursing has many unusual features, none the least being the different educational programs for becoming a nurse. Historical reasons account, in part, for some of the ways basic preparation for nursing has evolved, but a big factor has been the introduction of new educational systems in the country.

At this time, you may be a bit fuzzy about all this variety, wondering what the differences are in the programs, and even more important, which one is best for you. But a little fact-finding and soul-searching will give you the answers you seek.

FINDING YOUR NICHE IN NURSING

Why not ask nurses themselves their reasons for selecting a particular program? Some would make the same choice all over again while others might reconsider if they had all the proper information in the beginning. Listen to the following views from a few RNs, some you have met earlier.

A family nurse practitioner in Virginia, Dyan Aretakis selected a baccalaureate program because, "I expected greater autonomy and believed it would give me more of a chance for a supervisory role in the future and the ability to pursue graduate work."

Mary Jo Modica, a nurse manager at an Ohio medical center, reports that her first choice was also a baccalaureate in nursing. "After exploring different programs, I selected the BSN because I thought it would soon be the required entry level degree."

A desire "to enter the work force as quickly as possible" led Linda Anderson of Tennessee initially to a two-year associate degree program. She adds, however, that "after eight years of practice, I obtained my BSN, and seven years after that, an MSN. I realized that nursing was going to require further education to move ahead."

Tess H. Beltran, a staff nurse at a San Francisco medical center, received her diploma in the 1950s in the Philippines because "it was cheaper to enter a hospital program than the college/university program at that time." (Interestingly, her native Philippines now requires the baccalaureate as the entry level for nursing.)

The director of community affairs and education at the New York Regional Transplant Program, Miriam Perez began her career 20 years ago as an ADN graduate because the school was "local and less costly than other types of nursing programs." As the first-generation college student in her family, it represented an important achievement. A decade later, she earned her BSN because she wanted more knowledge as well as upward mobility. In the meantime, she married and had children. Enrolled in a master's degree nursing program, she declares: "Once you get into the academic community, you want to go on."

Two students who chose nontraditional entry level roads into nursing were Jennifer Biekert and Christine Cirlincione. Biekert, a 31-year-old graduate of the first doctor of nursing (ND) class at the University of Colorado in 1994, had a BS in Kinesiology (the study of the muscles of the body, the mechanics of motion). She was in a quandary about her future. She wanted to be involved in health care, but hadn't found her niche. When a secretary at the university's Health Sciences Center asked if she had looked into the exciting new nursing program there, she said: "I was instantly captivated by the vision of the program and jumped at the chance to enroll." She's now working in a walk-in primary care clinic for the students, staff, and faculty at the University of Denver, where she and three staff members see up to 80 patients a day.

72

Cirlincione, 26, a certified gerontological nurse practitioner in New Jersey, was a psychology major who decided she wanted to be a nurse. "I was interested in doing clinical work and wanted to work with patients on all levels, not just emotional health. But I didn't want to start from scratch!" So she selected Vanderbilt University's "bridge" program for those with non-nursing baccalaureates. After completing the prerequisites, she was able to earn her master's degree in a nursing specialty in two years.

WHICH PROGRAM IS BEST FOR YOU? CHECK THEM OUT

Are you fresh out of high school or do you have a few years to go? Or are you tempted to switch careers and change your working lifestyle? Nursing might be the career for you. Gone are the days when inflexibility was the hallmark of the nursing school. It's hard to believe that there was a time when men and married women were almost universally excluded from many programs. Today, however, the profession calls out for diversity, trying to woo men and women of all ages and ethnic backgrounds, the young and more mature, high school graduates, and second careerists.

Enrollments in nursing schools are on an upswing that reached an all-time high of 270,228 in 1993. Soaring enrollment figures, however, don't necessarily mean an increase in the number of nursing programs, but rather that acceptance at schools is becoming more competitive. These trends should imply one thing to you: you need to select the right nursing program and school, and make your selection soon.

Try not to be overwhelmed by the variety of choices. You will be able to narrow your decision by thoughtfully preparing for your future as a nurse. The key word here is "thoughtfully." You may begin by asking yourself several questions.

What Are My Long-Term Goals?

Reading about real-life nurses in previous chapters probably has your mind racing about the fascinating opportunities in the working environment. Which ones appealed to you? Have you already begun dreaming of becoming a critical care nurse, a staff nurse in ambulatory care, or a nurse in home health care? Or maybe you are setting your sights on becoming a clinical nurse specialist or nurse practitioner in some challenging area.

Each nursing education program prepares graduates for different opportunities. *Can I get there from here?* should be your question to determine which program can help you achieve your career goals. But don't worry if you still haven't figured out what your goals might be at this stage. You may need to gain more experience until it all comes together. Be patient.

Does Any One Program Appeal to Me More Than Others?

- *Maybe you see yourself as part of a college or university campus since you've always wanted to be part of the higher education scene.*
- *Maybe you've been out of school awhile and your study skills are rusty. Does a local community college seem a good place to test the waters?*
- *Maybe a relative or someone you admire graduated from a hospital school of nursing and you'd like to follow their lead.*

Can I Successfully Manage My Family Responsibilities While Attending School?

Returning to school certainly means quite a commitment on your part, but just think of the challenge in store for you while working toward your goal. At the same time, you probably have many other things going on in your life, like family and personal responsibilities. It is therefore important that you have the support of key people in your decision to become a nurse.

If you have children, you may wonder how to juggle the additional demands on your time. Have you figured out who will help with in-house child care or will you invest in day care outside the home? These are important considerations. Rest assured, however, you are not alone. Others have faced and overcome what may seem like obstacles and have reaped the rewards of their new profession.

How Much Time and Money Do I Want to Commit to School?

Undergraduate RN education programs vary from two to four or more years in most cases. How much time can you afford financially and personally? Have you figured out where the money will come from? Savings? Loans? Scholarships? As you'll see, funding resources are available to assist you.

In addition to concerns about financial aid, managing your time and personal obligations, and meeting your objectives, there must be a host of other questions that you'll want addressed before taking the big career plunge. Before firming up any perceptions, however, how about exploring the various entry-level nursing programs, checking out their unique features, and honing in on some of the newer trends in nontraditional education preparation.

THE BACCALAUREATE PROGRAM

Yearning for the ivy covered walls of academia? Programs leading to a bachelor of science in nursing (BSN) are mostly four years in length and affiliated with colleges or universities that offer the first professional degree in nursing. The popularity of the BSN program has grown dramatically in the past 30 years, with more than 500 baccalaureate programs today as compared to less than 200 in the 1960s.

What is special about BSN education? For starters, graduates of these programs acquire the groundwork leading to a college degree and for taking the licensure examination to become a registered nurse. Your education will be comparable to that of your peers in other disciplines. You'll be required to meet the general admission standards of the college and adhere to the same academic standards as students throughout the college and university.

The entire curriculum is challenging, with most programs offering the liberal arts and science courses during the first two years, followed by the nursing major in the upper division. The pre-nursing courses will generally include such subjects as biology, anatomy, physics, chemistry, physiology, English composition, a foreign language, sociology, psychology, nutrition, ethics, and business management.

Your nursing classes will focus on the promotion, maintenance, and restoration of the health of patients. Courses might include such subjects as basic and advanced concepts of nursing, medical and surgical care, mental health nursing, family and community health nursing, women's health, pharmacology, research methods, health problems in society, nursing process, social and professional issues and trends, nursing leadership, beginning research methods, and much more. Most BSN programs require at least 120 credits, including 58 or more credits in the nursing major.

The dynamic combination of education in science and humanities plus the experience gained from your academic and social life in a college or university setting truly differentiates a baccalaureate program from associate degree and hospital diploma programs. Whether you become involved in student government, write for your college newspaper, or join a caucus or club, you will meet and mix with students from other disciplines. Besides absorbing a rich cultural experience, you'll polish up your skills of communication, decision making, and negotiation which you will find indispensable in your practice.

This exceptional and varied background will help you develop the ability to think critically and apply your knowledge skillfully in the care of patients. You will learn to become a leader, teacher, and collaborator as well as a practitioner.

Another advantage is that only a BSN program prepares you in public health nursing through classwork and at clinical agencies. One innovative undergraduate program, for example, is at Northeastern University in Boston, MA. In 1990, the College of Nursing established a partnership with a medical school, 12 neighborhood health centers, and the city's Department of Health and Hospitals.

The goal was to provide community-based clinical experience for nursing and medical students. Students don't just practice within the walls of health centers, but undertake efforts involving local community agencies such as schools, housing projects, social services agencies, and others.

A bachelor of science in nursing is your springboard to the future. The program will prepare you to work in the widest range of health care settings and provide the foundation for graduate school that leads to professional tracks in advanced practice nursing, teaching, administration, research, and consultation. All this education, however, can mean greater expense than in other types of basic nursing programs. It goes without saying that the better prepared the faculty and the better the resources of the facility, the higher the cost of the program. Yet, in spite of the fact that BSN education is more costly in relation to time and money, keep in mind that the investment pays off in long-term mobility, recognition, and career advancement.

THE ASSOCIATE DEGREE NURSING PROGRAM

Pioneered in the early 1950s, the associate degree nursing program (ADN) became a part of one of the fastest growing educational movements in the nation—community and junior college preparation. By 1993, ADN programs reached the phenomenal number of 857. This type of nursing education often appeals to more mature students, particularly those with families who do not want to make long-term career commitments.

Associate degree programs have many positive features, but there are also limitations as with hospital diploma schools. As one of the fastest routes to RN licensure, AD education requires 18 months to two years of full-time study. A number of programs stipulate that science and general education courses be completed before a student can begin the nursing program. So, an ADN program might extend beyond the two years.

Located primarily in community or junior colleges, ADN programs are normally less expensive than those in senior colleges or universities. Another plus is that part-time study is encouraged to accommodate students with family and other responsibilities. Included in the curriculum are theory and supervised clinical learning along with some courses in the liberal arts and sciences. Graduates are prepared to practice in staff level positions, working in more structured environments such as hospitals and nursing homes.

The concept of associate degree nursing education was developed by Mildred Montag, a prominent nurse educator who envisioned a nurse with technical skills to provide direct patient care under the supervision of a professional (baccalaureate-prepared) nurse. She viewed the program as self-contained, with the graduate eligible to take the RN licensure examination.

Several changes in the original idea of ADN education have occurred in recent decades, although they have not been accepted by all nursing educators. Many students see the ADN as a first step in their education. As Anita Rogers, a student at Bergen County Community College explains, "I intend to go on for a BSN, but this way I can work and earn money while going back to school." This view, however, is in reality a long way around to becoming a professional nurse, particularly since the goals of ADN and baccalaureate education differ markedly. At the same time, there cannot be a lid placed on education.

ADN preparation is part of the system of higher education which awards college credit. If a graduate wishes to enter a baccalaureate program, the question of full or partial credit will depend on the admitting institution. Some BSN programs make it easier to go back to school by offering special entry routes for ADN graduates directly into baccalaureate and sometimes master's programs. The process by which a nurse with one credential advances to a higher level is called articulation.

The National League for Nursing, which accredits schools of nursing, supports diversified approaches to the transfer of academic credit between institutions and to the validation of prior extra-institutional learning. In a 1995 *Position Paper on Educational Mobility*, NLN urged nursing education programs to expand their present efforts to assure and promote educational mobility by providing articulation arrangements that have established policies for transferring of credits of graduates of ADN and diploma programs.

Is the ADN for you? If the overall length of your nursing education and money are important considerations, and your goal is to practice in structured settings such as hospitals and nursing homes, then the associate degree program might be your match.

THE HOSPITAL DIPLOMA PROGRAM

Long the mainstay of nursing education, hospital diploma programs, like their ADN counterparts, prepare graduates to work as beginning practitioners in acute, intermediate, ambulatory, and long-term health care settings. For many years, hospital-based diploma education was best described as "learning by doing," along with some classroom work, but mostly through providing nursing care within the hospital. Diploma preparation today, however, has evolved from an apprentice-type system to a stronger, formal educational program.

Even before nursing's push toward college and university-based education, hospital schools were beginning to decline in the 1960s. This trend resulted from the expense of running a hospital school and the cost to patients. Also, nursing students were expressing a desire for some type of collegiate education. In time, organized nursing's commitment to establish nursing education in schools of higher learning led many diploma schools to either close or phase into associate degree or baccalaureate programs. In 1993, 135 programs were operating.

Hospital diploma programs often appeal to more mature students because they offer a fast path to practice, generally two to three years. The hospital serves as the clinical facility, although many schools contract with other agencies or hospitals to provide a variety of clinical experiences for students.

Proponents of diploma education believe that the student's close relationship with the hospital develops a strong loyalty to nursing, in general, and specifically to hospital-based nursing. One disadvantage, however, is that a diploma is not an academic degree, and graduates who want to advance in their career will require more formal education. While programs exist that ease diploma grads into institutions of higher education, hospital schools of nursing are not chartered to grant degrees nor is credit automatically given for courses taken. Another problem concerns the complement of qualified faculty, since most nursing instructors prefer to teach in collegiate education.

If you wish to pursue nursing in a hospital diploma program, explore those schools offering a cooperative arrangement with a college or university offering courses for college credit. In this way, you'll have credits usually transferable if you decide to continue your education.

OTHER ENTRY LEVEL PROGRAMS PREPARING FOR RN LICENSURE

Already have a degree, but not in nursing? If you have your heart set on nursing, then you should know about special programs for people just like you—the nontraditional, second careerist, or second degree student.

Many schools welcome the second careerist. Studies have shown that these students are more likely to stay in school, have a greater interest in research, score higher on standardized tests and the licensing exam, and are more apt to pursue further education. The need for these second degree programs is real. One recent study reported a school with 380 applicants for 40 available slots!

One type of program allows the student with a non-nursing baccalaureate to earn a second baccalaureate (in nursing). These schools give credit for prior college education and offer advanced placement into the entry-level BSN program. A growing number of schools also offer accelerated coursework, and some even have special programs such as a calendar year of nursing courses, five days a week. It is often possible to complete an accelerated program in 1 to 1½ years of full-time study.

The Educational Program: Finding the Right Fit

For example, one East Coast university has an accelerated degree option for students with degrees in other fields that allows them to complete 58 credits in nursing in an intense 13-month program. Students must have completed the prerequisite courses and have a GPA of at least 3.0 or higher before they begin any nursing courses.

Another program for the second careerist offers an entry level degree in nursing at the master's level with a clinical specialty. Such programs are less common, but their numbers continue to grow. The "Bridge Program" at Vanderbilt University School of Nursing in Nashville, Tennessee, is a good example. Remember Chris Cirlincione, the former psychology major whom you met earlier in this chapter? Well, her nursing classmates in Vanderbilt's bridge program included two accountants, a lawyer, a pharmacist, a teacher, a counselor, a homemaker, and a fitness instructor. The average age was 35 years.

A non-nurse baccalaureate graduate with 72 transfer credits is eligible for the Vanderbilt program with direct entry and can complete the master of science in nursing (MSN) program in six semesters of full-time study. The bridge component of the curriculum consists of clinical and nonclinical courses containing beginning level nursing practice and content. Course sequence leads students from basic to advanced knowledge and skills levels, from less to more complex practice situations, and finally to specialist role preparation. The first three semesters of upper division generalist nursing courses do not end with a BSN, but "bridge" to the MSN program. In the last three semesters, the specialty master's component is offered.

Other schools offer second careerists the opportunity to pursue a master's degree while completing a BSN. At the University of Pennsylvania in Philadelphia, highly motivated, academically talented students may apply for admission to the undergraduate and graduate programs concurrently. They receive individualized programs based on their prior educational experience.

Another rare, but exciting educational choice for those with non-nursing degrees is the professional doctorate, the doctor of nursing (ND) degree. Although offered at the present time by only three universities, Case Western Reserve University in Cleveland, Rush University in Chicago, and the University of Colorado Health Sciences Center in Denver, the ND may be a trend worth watching in the near future. Following are descriptions of two of these extremely innovating programs.

According to director Sally Phillips, the ND program at the University of Colorado offers an entry-level degree to the profession, preparing graduates for clinical practice as a broad-based practitioner across the life span of clients. ND graduates are generally expected to have the ability to function in complex situations and to collaborate with other health care professionals in a variety of health care settings. They practice as generalists or go on to specialize through certification, or to obtain master's degrees in a clinical specialty. The university graduated its first class in 1993 with 10 students.

What kind of student does this type of program draw? Phillips says her program "doesn't attract shy people! Applicants are risk takers, entrepreneurial types who are expected to make their own way." ND candidates, by and large, usually have varied backgrounds with degrees and life experience in teaching, other health disciplines, research, or business.

Admission requirements to the University of Colorado Nurse Doctorate Program are the same as to the MD (doctor of medicine) or DDS (doctor of dental science) programs—a college degree or 120 credits from a college or university. The four-year curriculum (114 credits) includes summers, and covers clinical sciences, clinical arts, and humanities, discipline-specific human caring nursing, and health professional and ethical foundations. Students are eligible to take the RN licensure examination after completing two years of study. The fourth year is a full-time clinical residency program as a licensed nurse at a sponsored site throughout the state.

Similar to Colorado's ND program, Case Western Reserve University also prepares non-nurse college graduates. The course runs for four years and prepares students for licensure as an RN during the first two years. In the remaining period, the focus is on clinical practice as a nurse midwife or nurse practitioner in such specialties as adult, family, pediatric, gerontological, psychiatric-mental health, or women's health.

WHAT ABOUT MY CLINICAL EXPERIENCE?

Once you've made the decision to begin your educational program, you can expect lots of classwork. Back to the books, lectures, note taking, term papers, examinations, and, of course, burning the proverbial midnight oil. But you will take it all in stride because of the exciting world of nursing that is in store for you.

From the beginning, you probably have one compelling thought: "When am I going to take care of my first patient?" That big step may occur sooner than you think, but your instructor will ensure that you and your classmates will be ready for your introduction to the clinical area.

Regardless of your nursing program, you will have opportunities to observe and participate in the planning of patient care. You will have diverse experiences in a variety of health care agencies and settings, where your role will be to learn and not to work. Traditional sites of clinical learning include hospitals and medical centers, clinics, nursing homes, social service organizations, health maintenance organizations, and other settings.

Many schools also try to select nontraditional types of experiences so that students can be exposed to such populations as the homeless, prison inmates, substance abusers, and AIDS patients.

When assigned for clinical experience in one field, there may be a preconference to discuss objectives and projected outcomes, such as learning a procedure or developing a skill like changing a dressing or giving a bath. A postconference will evaluate your performance. In colleges or universities, there may be separate clinical instructors or your faculty might have practice privileges and carry a patient load at the clinical practice site. In addition to teaching, this faculty member would normally accompany you for the learning experience. Many students like this arrangement because they feel "at home" on the clinical unit with the instructor serving as a role model.

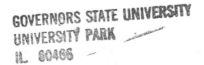

While every school is different and the type and amount of time spent in clinical experience will vary, rest assured that a good program will see that you gain the necessary skills and knowledge. To make students comfortable in the clinical setting, some schools encourage them to spend extra time in study labs, while others offer special clinical concentrations at the end of the program that simulate job situations as closely as possible. Your school might even set up summer, paid work-study programs or a supervised clinical practicum.

The *preceptorship* is another extracurricular clinical avenue. A one-on-one experience with a clinical expert, a preceptorship can be a mix of classwork and hands-on practice. These normally unpaid opportunities help you learn additional skills through a give-and-take relationship with your preceptor as a role model. As a new RN, you might work for a hospital that offers preceptorships or internships for new graduates. (Chapter 8 discusses these types of programs in more detail.)

Another way to gain clinical experience is to locate a hospital that offers *externships,* which are paid positions, often as a full-time summer job. Externships may be offered through your clinical facility, but normally are not considered part of your curriculum.

If you are fortunate, you may also find a mentor as a student or a graduate nurse. Most successful people have mentors, older, more experienced nurses who act as voluntary, caring counselors, advisors, teachers, and guides throughout your early career. Mentors help you make career decisions, steer your course for greater job satisfaction, and help prepare you for leadership roles. In time, when you become a seasoned professional, you may begin to nurture a promising young student yourself.

THE PRACTICAL NURSING PROGRAM

Licensed Practical Nurses (LPNs) are often referred to as Licensed Vocational Nurses (LVNs) in some states. They are auxiliary workers who practice under the supervision of registered nurses. Most

LPNs work in structured settings, such as hospitals (21 percent), long-term care facilities (30 percent), and in the home. They receive their preparation usually in a 12-month program located in public vocational and technical schools, high schools, hospitals, community colleges, and a variety of health care agencies. On completing the course, they are eligible to take the licensing examination for practical nursing.

The program stresses technical skills and direct patient care, but offers only a limited foundation in the social and physical sciences. Many LPNs continue to demonstrate their desire to become RNs. In 1992, close to 25 percent of all RN graduates first practiced as LPNs. At present, some ADN and BSN programs provide "ladders" to enable the licensed practical nurse to advance to RN status in an organized process, but they are not as common as articulation programs for ADN and diploma graduates to advance to BSN programs. Although the practical nursing program is brief and normally inexpensive, the salary potential, status, and advancement opportunities are limited.

ALREADY AN RN?

Although it is more cost effective in the long run to select the right nursing program from the beginning, it may not always be possible. After they have been in practice a while, some nurses discover that they want to pursue new roles or higher level positions which will require further knowledge and skills. If that describes you, it means back to school for more education.

There are numerous *RN completion programs* across the country that provide articulation programs to assist those RNs who want more education. Various mechanisms are used to validate knowledge, such as transfer credits, challenge exams, and tests of clinical skills in learning laboratories. It is even possible for an RN with a diploma or associate degree to earn a BSN en route to the MSN. At the University of Texas Health Science Center in San Antonio, a flexible system enables qualified RNs to meet the requirements for the master's degree in five semesters of full-time study. On completing the program, the student receives a BSN and MSN simultaneously.

Another option for RNs who want to go back to school is *the self-paced program,* in which students establish their own pattern using self-study, computers, and multimedia. Flexibility is the watchword as long as they meet the requirements set by the degree-granting institution. Regents College, The University of the State of New York, Albany, is the only National League for Nursing accredited, self-paced external degree BSN program now available. Students must earn a total of 120 semester credits, including 48 nursing credits documented by standardized examinations.

The Regents College program has one major difference from its conventional campus-bound cousins. No classroom instruction! Rather, RC issues the degree requirements and study materials, leaving it up to the student to demonstrate knowledge learned through approved examinations and other evaluation processes. Since the program was established in the early 1970s, there have been more than 10,000 ADN and 3,000 BSN graduates. Self-study programs, however, may not be suitable for everyone. Successful candidates must be highly motivated, persistent, independent, and willing to accept the challenge of self-directed study.

MAKING THE PERFECT MATCH

Remember, your personal needs and career goals should determine the program and school that is your best match. Of course, your objectives may change after you enter the nursing program and even later on after you are in practice. But you probably have an inkling of the kind of nursing role and practice setting you see for yourself as well as the type of program you need to achieve your goals. At this point, you are ready for that awesome task of narrowing your choices of nursing schools.

Catalogs, the old standby, are still the most effective way to check out specific schools since they contain a vast amount of valuable information. You'll want to call or write to all the schools whose programs you want to consider. The catalogs should give you the background and history of your prospective school as well as the philosophy of the nursing program. They will spell out expenses for tuition, as well as mandatory fees and cost estimates for books and supplies. Financial aid opportunities and requirements will be outlined, as well as application procedures.

The catalog will explain the programs of study and degree requirements and detail the curriculum set up. You'll also find descriptions of the types of courses you'll take, the names and credentials of the faculty, and a list of the health care facilities affiliated with the school. Also look for descriptions of academic resources, such as clinical skills and computer laboratories, the library and on-line databases, or other learning centers.

Most catalogs will also discuss the campus location, student life, school policies, and characteristics of the nursing student population. And, of course, you will find specific admission requirements and prerequisites.

Another resource is *Peterson's Guide to Nursing Programs,* (published annually) available in most libraries. It lists detailed information about baccalaureate and graduate nursing programs accredited by the National League for Nursing. Published in cooperation with the American Association of Colleges of Nursing, the guide provides geographic school profiles and an excellent section on in-depth descriptions voluntarily prepared by individual schools of nursing.

The National League for Nursing Center for Career Advancement can also help. For a fee, it will do a customized computer search of its extensive national database to help you match your needs to specific nursing programs. The Center offers quick access to reliable career and continuing education information. You can request a customized search of undergraduate, graduate and specialty practitioner programs, and practical nursing programs. Contact the NLN Center for Career Advancement at 1-800-669-9656, extension 145 to order a search.

Finally, if you have a computer and modem, you might also find information by tapping into one of the available computer databases available through various on-line services such as America On-Line® or Compuserve®.

WHAT COMES NEXT? GET PERSONAL!

Once you zero in on a few schools, it's time to make personal contact. Check out the catalog to find out how to schedule a visit to the school. Your contact may be an admissions officer (in the nursing school), the student affairs department, an academic program director, or perhaps the office of the dean or chair of the nursing program. But every school will be different.

While visiting the campus, try to set up a meeting to talk with a student or graduate of the school. He or she can give you valuable insights and explain the pros and cons of the school from a student perspective. Give yourself plenty of time to observe the campus and the facilities you will be using, such as dormitories, clinical laboratories, classrooms, and the library. Can you "see" yourself studying there?

As you begin to check out nursing schools, stay as organized as possible. Make lists of questions, take notes, and write down the answers. This isn't the time to trust your memory. You will find that your notes provide a perfect way to refresh your memory when you sit down to make your final choices.

Wait, did we say questions? What kind? What's important? Here are some basics to think about as you peruse catalogs and other sources and talk to students and faculty. But be sure to add your own.

What is the nature of the curriculum? What kinds of nursing courses does the school offer? What is the philosophy of the nursing program? Check out the names and credentials of the school's faculty. What is the percentage of faculty with doctorates? Who knows, you might even be lucky enough to find a famous name as the chair or dean of your nursing program. Remember you'll take courses offered by departments other than the nursing school, so look them over and the faculty as well.

What are the admission requirements? Most schools require an undergraduate grade point average of at least 3.0. You'll probably have to submit scores from one of the standardized tests such as the Scholastic Aptitude Test (SAT). Also, you might have to complete a list of prerequisite courses as well. Expect to submit letters of recommendation and possibly a written personal essay. Many schools also request a personal interview. Lastly, some health history documentation is frequently required.

Is the school accredited by the National League for Nursing? You've probably heard that accreditation is important when referring to nursing programs, and that is true. State-approval of nursing schools, required by law, ensures minimum standards. Increasing numbers of schools, however, also seek voluntary accreditation by the National League for Nursing because it represents higher standards for educational quality and accountability. NLN's criteria are determined by the collective thinking of national experts.

If you are eventually interested in graduate school, the military, or military reserves, only graduates of NLN-accredited schools of nursing can apply for acceptance. "I plan to get my master's and doctorate," one student observed, "and I can't afford to make any mistakes. I looked only at NLN-accredited schools."

Can I afford this school? You will be more successful in financing your nursing education by starting your search early. Begin with the schools you wish to attend. Most financial aid comes from the school itself which administers federal and state funds as well as school or university scholarships. The United States Department of Education reports that 80 percent of all student aid comes from federal and state programs.

Almost all government assistance is based on student need although some merit-based programs exist. Your need is determined by computing the cost of tuition, mandatory fees, and other expenses compared to your income or family assets. Financial aid based on merit is awarded for outstanding academic achievement and other special qualifications set by the grantor.

Contact the school's financial aid office for information. Be prepared to fill out a need-analysis form to demonstrate how much you or your family can contribute to your education. A school can compute a financial aid package putting together a mix of federal, state, and private sources.

Financial aid takes several forms: a *scholarship or grant*, a contribution that does not need to be paid back; a *fellowship*, a grant for study in graduate education that does not need to be paid back; and a *loan*, which needs to be repaid, often with interest. *Work study programs* allow students to work and earn money for school. *Traineeships* are federal stipends and tuition grants which do not have to be repaid.

You'll want to explore local, state, regional, and national sources and look for money from special sources, both private and governmental. Be sure to review NLN's handy resource, *Scholarships and Loans for Nursing Education*. Updated each year, it outlines available scholarships and loans, as well as special aid for minority students.

If you have other questions than those addressed above, jot them down for future reference. No question can be considered unimportant when information is needed for making a serious career decision.

Once you have selected your nursing program and found several schools that particularly interest you, you have already taken that first big step. It's a good idea to pick at least three schools and apply to all of them to increase your chances of acceptance. Nursing schools are very competitive. Stay on the right track and you will achieve your goal to become a registered nurse.

*　*　*

The opening of the Nightingale schools in America represented a dramatic new chapter in the history of nursing. As you have seen, nursing education has moved progressively over the years into the college and university system. This phenomenon has been triggered by the need to keep pace with the profession's expanding scope of practice and to meet the challenges of health care toward the end of this century and into the next.

Nursing school will be a personal and intellectual challenge as you master nursing theory, sciences, and technology. Your logical, well-informed decision about the type of nursing program and the school you select will serve you well as you prepare for your new career.

8

Graduation: The Big Moment and What Comes Next

Believe it or not, in a few years you'll be a graduate nurse (GN) proudly holding your hard earned degree or diploma and eager to get on with your career. Graduation, however, is only the first step toward achieving your career goal. Next you must become licensed by your state's board of nursing, which administers the National Council Licensure Examination (NCLEX).

THE NEW LOOK IN NURSING LICENSURE

How did this come about? First, it's important to know that your profession is regulated by state law which protects the public by setting standards for entry into the profession and for removing unqualified practitioners. These laws or nursing practice acts define the practice of nursing and describe the scope of nursing practice in a state.

Who are the players in this process? Each state has an agency, usually called a board of nursing, holding the power to issue, renew, revoke, and suspend licenses for professional and practical nurses, to grant reciprocity for nurses licensed in other states, and to set continuing education requirements for relicensure. Without state approval, a school cannot operate, and graduates are ineligible to take the licensure examination. Overseeing the licensing examination is the National Council of State Boards of Nursing, which works in conjunction with the Educational Testing Service (ETS).

In 1994, nursing licensure entered the computer age through Computer Adaptive Testing (CAT). The examination differs markedly from the "pencil-and-paper" test of earlier years when every candidate took the same written examination on the same days.

CAT is given nationally at an ETS Testing Center or at one of 200+ Sylvan Technology Centers. There's at least one location, maybe more, in your state or territory. You can schedule appointments at your convenience, 15 hours a day, six days a week (even Sundays during peak demands), making the test as hassle free as possible.

Computer adaptive testing is a unique process that individualizes each examination. As you answer correctly, the computer, which knows the difficulty of all 3,000 questions in the program, selects more difficult ones while it checks your competency against the level required to pass the examination. When you reach the point at which the computer judges you have passed (or that you have failed), the examination ends. CAT's goal aims to determine your competency based on the difficulty of the questions you can answer correctly, not on the number of correct answers.

You will receive the results in three or four weeks. Statistics indicate that between 85 and 93 percent of first-time, U.S.-educated candidates pass the exam.

GETTING READY FOR NCLEX

The NCLEX examination is one of the most important tests you will take in becoming a nurse. Keep in mind, however, that you have time to prepare between graduation and the scheduling of the test.

How are your study skills? Those good ones you developed in school should serve you well as you review for the NCLEX. Bone up on any difficult content areas. If help is needed, there are ways to assist in preparation. You'll find out about several review groups by reading nursing journals, participating in student organizations, and attending conventions and job fairs. There are also review texts, review and preparatory skill guides and test-taking guides, review courses of various lengths, audio cassettes, and computer assisted instruction from associations, independent companies, and publishers. The National Council provides several videotapes to introduce CAT, walking you through the testing experience.

Hundreds of schools of nursing and hospitals have purchased the National League for Nursing's *RN Computer Challenge*. This study/learning software helps NCLEX candidates drill and practice in a colorful, fun, game environment. After responding to questions, players see the correct answer and its rationale.

Some of the resource materials will give hints to improve your test-taking and study skills, but don't expect them to teach you nursing content. They will, however, help you pinpoint your strengths and weaknesses. A thorough self-evaluation plus a selection of up-to-date review materials can increase the probability of your success on the licensure examination.

BEFORE YOU KNOW IT, YOU'LL BE AN RN

Say hello to the real world. The good news is that the overwhelming majority of new nurses find jobs either before or right after graduation, a good reason for being attracted to nursing in the first place.

As noted earlier, you'll probably start your career as a general duty or staff nurse in a hospital. Hospitals can vary greatly depending on geographic location, size, whether they are private or public, or by specialty. Regardless of where your first job is, you probably will feel a bit skittish in your new role. Just think back to how awkward you felt when learning to drive, ride a bicycle, or roller skate. You had the skills, but lacked the experience to feel sure of yourself. Your transition from student to RN may be a little like that.

In school, you have been in a controlled environment under the watchful eye of an instructor, but now you are entering the world of patient care. Being a student in a clinical learning situation is one thing, but as a graduate in the same setting it can look and feel quite different. The only difference, however, is that your status has changed. Yet, no one expects you to adjust immediately; there are people and systems to help you. It won't take long to learn what's expected in the employment setting and to feel a part of your new environment.

MAKING THE TRANSITION

You can ease the transition into your first job in a number of ways. Of course it is natural to have some anxiety, but try to communicate a confident attitude. Act and look professional, and be yourself—that's probably the best advice. People will know you are new, but it's up to you to show a willingness to learn and listen. Also, your sense of humor will go a long way. We all need to learn to laugh at ourselves a little.

Your employer wants you to succeed. Some facilities offer *clinical preceptorships* for graduate nurses, those one-on-one experiences with a staff nurse. Others might have an *internship* program to help graduate nurses ease into the work force. The internships usually combine traditional job orientation information with supervised experience within the area of the hospital where the new RN will be employed. They are usually slated for a specific period of time during which the graduate receives less pay.

You can expect your new employer to offer some type of formal orientation program for new graduates where you'll learn about the facility, its philosophy, policies and procedures, and the equipment, supplies, and other information. Most of all, you will discover what is expected of you as a practicing nurse in the institution. So, when considering a prospective employer, look at the orientation process. How long is it for new staff? How is it structured? Is the orientation individualized?

You will also want to know if an evaluation process exists throughout the orientation. In addition, does further orientation occur on the specialty unit or when transferring between units or shifts? Often, the program matches new employees with the clinical area where they will be working.

Don't forget about mentoring, which was mentioned earlier. As support persons, mentors can be helpful with a broad range of professional and personal issues and especially in the transition from graduate nurse to registered nurse. While the experienced person usually initiates the relationship, don't be reluctant to be on the lookout for persons with whom you feel comfortable and whom you admire. Ask them for advice and suggestions.

A final tip: Think of your first job as another nursing class where you'll learn all the things you didn't pick up in nursing school. Surveys show that after one year in the labor force, the majority of newly licensed nurses are content working in nursing and happy with their present job situation, mostly in hospital nursing. Don't be discouraged if it takes months to make a smooth transition. Rest assured, as time passes, you will be more in control.

WHAT ARE YOUR OPTIONS
FOR THE FUTURE?

No matter how much you like your job, eventually you may get a yen for a different type of position or for more responsibility. Educational standards for nursing are on the upswing, and most nursing leaders know that to advance in the profession, you will need at the very least a bachelor's degree. So whether you're an associate degree nurse who wants a BSN or a baccalaureate nurse who wants to become a clinical specialist, it means returning to campus life for more formal study (see Figure 8.1).

Fortunately, nursing education programs are more flexible today than ever before. Few nursing leaders view any degree as "terminal," but rather recognize the need for lifelong education. You already know how nursing programs provide articulation from one to another. The ability to move along in an organized fashion, advancing to different levels of nursing education, is often referred to as a "career ladder," "career mobility," or "vertical mobility."

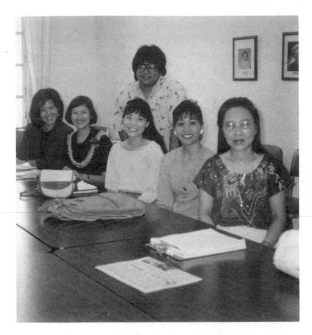

Figure 8.1 Professor Aurora Villafuerte (second from left) with her nursing students during a seminar at University of Hawaii, in 1991.

All these terms imply that you can change your goals and find the right rung on the career ladder. Nursing values education as well as experience, providing an innovative approach to accommodate the learning and career needs of students. While more education may seem to be a million miles down the road at this time, the chances are that one day you will be seeking it. Perhaps you will consider graduate education.

MOVING UP ON THE EDUCATION LADDER

It's truly an exciting time to enter nursing. Graduate education in nursing is on the fast track. In the 1950s, fewer than 1,500

RNs held master's degrees in nursing. Today, more than 30,000 students are enrolled in master's programs in 252 schools. There are several tracks to pursue, although many RNs want to go the route of advanced practice nursing. A whopping 44 percent of graduations in 1993 were from clinical specialist practice programs and 25 percent from nurse practitioner programs. Even in the rough and tumble climate of health care reform, graduate programs are growing as nurses prepare for challenging and innovative clinical roles.

Advanced practice appeals to nurses for a variety of reasons, and in time it might tempt you, too. RNs with these skills usually have greater freedom and independence in their practice. As a nurse with a master's degree, you'll command a higher salary and have greater opportunities for career growth. You'll be dazzled by the variety of master's level clinical specialties. Among the four advanced practice roles are the Nurse Practitioner (NP), Clinical Nurse Specialist (CNS), Certified Nurse Midwife (CNM), and Certified Nurse Anesthetist (CRNA). Comprising the curriculum are clinical and didactic components related to a nursing specialty as well as professional certification. While some nurses have been practicing in these roles without a master's degree, they have been "grandfathered" into the designation. For the future, however, a minimum of a master's degree will be required.

Loretta Ford, who founded the nurse practitioner movement, is encouraged by the significant contributions of NPs. Recently, she commented about her dream for professional nursing and nurses that, in part, came true. "Not just because of me," Ford declared, "but because a small band of courageous and clinically competent nurse practitioners took up the torch that the pediatric nurse practitioner ignited. They changed the world of nursing and health care."

In 1993, master's degree programs for nurse practitioners totalled 136, and the number continues to grow. NPs provide primary health care in ambulatory settings, inpatient hospitals, community clinics, health maintenance organizations, long-term care facilities, physicians' offices, and other sites. They handle a wide range of physical and mental health problems, prescribe medication in most states, diagnose and treat health problems, and stress health promotion and prevention. The most sought after practice is in family health, followed by pediatrics, adult health, and gerontology. For the more than 50,000 nurse practitioners, salaries on average come to more than $40,000 a year.

Clinical Nurse Specialists are expert practitioners with a master's degree in a clinical specialty such as oncology, adult or child-psychiatric-mental health, community health, medical-surgical nursing, critical care, and maternal and child nursing among others. Salaries for the almost 60,000 CNSs can vary from $30,000 up to $80,000 depending on specialty and geographic location. CNSs can be found in small rural hospitals as well as large teaching facilities, in clinics, industry, and often in their own practice. Adult health/medical-surgical is the most popular specialty.

Nurse practitioners and clinical nurse specialists emerged during the late 1960s. Recently, some blurring of their roles has occurred, with the trend toward NPs working in acute care institutions as well as in the community. In the early 1990s, the American Nurses Association merged its Councils of NPs and CNSs into a unified Council of Nurses in Advanced Practice.

Certified Registered Nurse Anesthetists (CRNAs), numbering 24,000, may legally administer anesthesia in all 50 states without the supervision of an anesthesiologist. CRNAs administer more than 65 percent of the 26 million anesthetics given to patients annually in the United States and are the sole providers of anesthesia in 85 percent of rural hospitals.

The position of the American Association of Nurse Anesthetists (AANA) is that after January 1998, all nurse anesthesia programs must be at the master's or higher level. At present, several universities in the nation offer master's and doctoral programs preparing nurse anesthetists.

Certified Nurse Midwives provide family-centered health care to women, including gynecological care to well women and low-risk obstetrical care in clinics, birthing centers, and homes. The approximately 6,000 CNMs earn an average salary of more than $43,600. They practice in clinics, private offices, hospitals, birthing centers, or in the woman's home.

MORE ABOUT GRADUATE EDUCATION

Graduate programs grant a variety of nursing degrees, including the MS, MSN, MA, MPHN, and EdM. In addition to advanced clinical practice, master's level education prepares nurses for leadership roles in teaching and administration. A number of schools offer dual degrees with graduate programs in business, law, public health, and other areas. A popular type of joint program offers an MSN/MBA degree, which prepares nurse administrators for top level management positions. Candidates study financial and operations management, marketing, accounting, economics, management, and other related courses.

Entrance requirements for master's degree programs in nursing vary according to the institution, but normally require RN licensure, graduation from an NLN-accredited baccalaureate nursing program, a GPA of 3.0 or higher, college transcripts, letters of reference, satisfactory completion of the Graduate Record Examination (GRE) or Millers Analogies Test (MAT), and one or more years of work experience. A personal interview may also be required.

The curriculum will include advanced courses in the study area plus supervised field experience or a practicum for clinical, administrative, or teaching majors. You may be required to prepare a thesis, although some programs suggest an independent project in its place. Most full-time graduate programs are one to two years long, requiring a minimum of 30 to 45 credits. For example, at the Frances Payne Bolton School of Nursing, Case Western Reserve University, Cleveland, the MSN program requires 40 semester hours of study for a Nurse Practitioner specialty, nurse midwifery, or nurse anesthesia. The majority of RNs, however, study part time with 75 percent following this pattern in 1993. Some schools offer flexible nontraditional programs, such as "summer only," off campus, exchange programs between institutions, and one day a week classes.

Reaching your master's degree on the career ladder is a victory that brings prestige, satisfaction, higher salary, and job mobility. But what's available for those who reach for doctoral education, the top rung of the ladder? Although post-master's education may not be for everyone, the future is extremely bright for those who go for it. Doctoral nursing education has come a long way, since before the mid-1940s when a nurse who wanted a doctorate had to earn it in a field outside of nursing. Today, 54 schools award doctorates, including the doctor of philosophy, doctor of nursing science, doctor of science in nursing, and doctor of education.

Generally, the PhD is viewed as a degree that emphasizes developing theory and basic research, while the clinical doctorate, the doctor of nursing science, aims to use theory and engage in applied research. Whatever kind of doctoral degree nurses earn, they are expected to be qualified for teaching, research, and administration.

The changes in nursing practice and the growth of nursing education in institutions of higher education have also affected the supply and demand for qualified teachers. The issue is not merely the faculty shortage but the *shortage of faculty educated as teachers in addition to their clinical knowledge.*

Doctoral programs are normally the equivalent of three years of full-time study, but approximately 60 percent of doctoral students study part time while pursuing their career. Admission requirements vary, normally requiring a master's degree from an NLN-accredited school, RN licensure, GRE or MAT scores, clinical experience, letters of reference, and transcripts.

Too early to think about a doctorate? Probably, but listen to the story of Eileen O'Neill, an associate professor at the University of Massachusetts at Dartmouth, who earned her PhD in 1992. She didn't start out expecting to teach. "It was an accident, like most of life," she explains. After working as a head nurse on a hectic medical unit, however, with a crew of young staff nurses under her, a colleague noticed how well she guided them and planted the seed in her mind. Later, after deciding to attain her master's degree ("I didn't know enough!"), she eased into teaching.

O'Neill enjoys watching her students grow and develop professional attitudes and behavior. "It's great," she says. Until a few years ago, she did clinical practice every summer, but her teaching, research, publishing, and speaking engagements now take up most of her time. She firmly believes in nursing faculty having a broad knowledge base and strong clinical skills.

100

Graduation: The Big Moment and What Comes Next

Although reaching the top of your formal career ladder may be many years away, plan ahead. Someday, you may want to conduct research, teach in a university, or be a dean at a school of nursing or a top level administrator. A doctorate in nursing will be the best ticket to your future.

*   *   *

Right now, just getting accepted to nursing school and graduating is all you can think about, but don't sell yourself short. The closest distance between you and your goals is a deliberate, straight line. Be aware of all your options. You have an exciting new career at your fingertips. The wide world of nursing is just a few years away.

9

The Voyage Ahead:
Becoming a Professional

Once you graduate from nursing school, become licensed, and join the work force, you're a professional. Right? Yes and No on both counts. Sure, you have the credentials, but professionalism doesn't end there. Professionals never stop satisfying their thirst for knowledge. You will want to consider continuing education, certification, participating in professional organizations, keeping up with the nursing literature, and publishing reports of innovative ideas and research.

CONTINUING EDUCATION:
THE INFORMAL ROUTE

Staying abreast of clinical techniques and technologies, issues, and trends in the profession will be an ongoing process throughout your career. That's where continuing education (CE) comes in. It promotes professional development and advances the career goals of the nurse.

Why is continuing education important? Because it will build on your educational background and experience, enhancing your area of practice (clinical or otherwise) to the end of maintaining and improving the health of the public. CE is based on previously acquired knowledge, skills, and attitudes, helping you to maintain and increase your competence, while fostering personal and professional growth. RN learners participate in identifying their own needs and seek CE activities to meet them.

About a third of state boards of nursing recommend mandatory continuing education for license renewal. Almost all require CE courses for nurses applying to reenter clinical practice, but there are variations from state to state. Renewal requirements are usually between 10 to 15 contact hours a year (a contact hour is 50 minutes in an approved learning experience). At present, a few states even target specific subjects for CE credit for licensure renewal. New York, for example, requires courses in child abuse and infectious disease control.

Most employers provide funding and time off for continuing education as an employee benefit. Opportunities abound throughout the country through colleges, hospitals, professional organizations, nursing journals, self-study courses, computer-assisted instruction, and more. To ensure quality, CE providers should be accredited by the American Nurses Credentialing Center or by a state board of nursing.

YOU UNDERSTAND CE, BUT WHAT ABOUT CERTIFICATION?

Perhaps you've heard of certification before, for example, the expression "board-certified physicians," often referred to as diplomates. Most other professions also have certification programs, including nursing, which joined the ranks with its early efforts in the 1970s. Remember some of the nurses you met in earlier chapters? One thing they had in common was certification in their area of expertise.

So why is being certified important? Isn't it enough to have a good education and be licensed? Both good questions. The best answer is that certification demonstrates a nurse's specialized knowledge and skills. Unlike licensure, a once-in-a-lifetime test of minimal competency, certification is a voluntary, peer review process that promotes competency, visibility, marketability, and quality among practitioners, and shows continued professional growth. It also signals to the public and your employer that you have taken an extra step to demonstrate your commitment to giving high-quality care.

When you graduate from your basic nursing program, you are considered a *generalist*, prepared to work in your clinical area of choice. In time, you might qualify to take a certification examination, but your status as a generalist working on a specialty unit remains the same. Only nurses with advanced formal preparation can be certified as *specialists*. Although both groups may carry the designation of certified nurses, there is a marked difference in the scope of their responsibilities.

Almost 200,000 RNs are certified, but the standards vary considerably among the specialty certification boards. That is why the American Board of Nursing Specialties (ABNS) was established in 1991 to promote consistency and encourage uniformity in standards and requirements for achieving certification. Among the organizations that offer certification, 12 have been accepted into the ABNS.

When you're ready, certification is worth the extra effort. Certified RNs command higher salaries, have better job prospects, and more job mobility.

GETTING INVOLVED IN
PROFESSIONAL ORGANIZATIONS

Many nurses find participating in voluntary activities rewarding. They share their experience by working with professional organizations or local groups, such as the American Red Cross, by volunteering at clinics, or serving as advisers to nursing student organizations or future nursing clubs. Nurses are also involved in consumer health education programs such as health fairs and health teaching classes.

Association membership enriches you as a professional. Joining a nursing organization opens doorways to network with your colleagues, obtain continuing education and certification opportunities, develop leadership skills, keep informed of trends and issues affecting the profession, and to mentor and support others. Associations give you a sense of community within your profession and also provide the clout, for example, to bring about legislative or policy changes. And don't forget that the visibility you get can help advance your career. You get all these benefits, plus the fun of being part of the action.

Attending the group's national convention, a thrilling professional shot in the arm, is one of the most attractive features of being an active association member. Imagine making new friends from across the country, attending stimulating meetings, learning about cutting-edge technologies or techniques, hearing dynamic speakers, often nursing leaders who you have heard or read about, or debating and voting on your association's policies as a delegate. Many conventions have trade shows with hundreds of exhibitors—from nurse recruiters and book and journal publishers to pharmaceutical companies and equipment manufacturers. Since national groups rotate convention sites around the nation, attendance allows you to combine professional activities and personal travel.

The number of nursing organizations is exploding, with more than 100 of all types and sizes. The first nursing organization you'll probably come across as a student is the **National Student Nurses' Association** (NSNA) through one of its school and state chapters. Founded in 1953, the NSNA is the only national organization for undergraduate nursing students, drawing members from state-approved schools leading to licensure as an RN. Students join NSNA directly, paying a combination of national and state dues. They receive numerous membership benefits, including a subscription to *Imprint,* the association's official magazine. The NSNA Foundation administers a scholarship program that distributes thousands of dollars annually to members and others.

NSNA nurtures professionalism and helps students to understand the importance of association work, giving opportunities to test leadership skills at the school, state, and national levels. Today, you will find many nursing leaders who were active in NSNA as students.

The **American Nurses Association** (ANA), founded in 1896, is a federation of state nursing organizations. As the national professional organization for registered nurses, its priorities focus on the needs of individual nurses and the public they serve. You'll want to join the more than 200,000 nurses belonging to ANA when you begin your practice. Nurses become members through a state or territorial organization rather than directly through ANA.

As the spokesperson for the profession, ANA works for the improvement of health standards and the availability of health care services for all people, fosters high standards of nursing, stimulates the professional development of nurses, and advances their economic and general welfare. It also establishes a code of ethical conduct for nurses, ensures a system of credentialing in nursing, and initiates and influences legislation and health policy.

ANA's legislative activities are of major importance. Located in Washington, DC, the association represents nursing on major issues affecting the profession including funds for nursing education, health care reform, and issues related to the quality of care. The association is well respected for its nationwide grassroots network and for its behind-the-scenes as well as visible lobbying efforts on nursing's behalf.

A political triumph for ANA and all other major nursing organizations came in June 1993 when the National Center for Nursing Research (NCNR) was given a more prominent status within the National Institutes of Health as the National Institute of Nursing Research (NINR). NCNR had been established in 1985, but after intense lobbying efforts by nursing organizations and nurses across the country, the Institute was launched. The victory gave nursing research the visibility and credibility it deserved.

ANA-PAC, the American Nurses Association Political Action Committee, educates nurses about health issues and encourages participation in the political process. And nurses are involved! In fact, an ANA survey showed that 91 percent of state nurses association members are registered to vote, 75 percent have written a letter to a politician giving their opinion, and 58 percent have made political contributions. ANA-PAC also supports political candidates by endorsement or monetary contributions.

ANA's research arm, the American Nurses Foundation, founded in the 1950s, solicits, receives, and/or administers funds for a number of projects. Grants have sponsored activities in such areas as HIV prevention, managed care, and managing genetic information. The American Nurses Credentialing Center (ANCC) is a separately incorporated organization through which the ANA serves its own credentialing programs. ANCC certifies nurses and accredits organizations using ANA standards of nursing practice, nursing services, and continuing education.

The association is also the sole stockholder in the independent American Journal of Nursing Company, which publishes *The American Journal of Nursing* and several other journals and assembles an active video and film service. *AJN* magazine is ANA's professional journal, while *The American Nurse* goes to all members as the official newspaper.

The **National League for Nursing** (NLN), whose roots go back to 1893, is comprised of registered nurses, professionals from related fields, interested lay persons, agencies involved in nursing education and service, and community groups. NLN's original charter defines the organization's purpose "that the nursing needs of the people will be met." Membership is either individual or through an agency. NLN sets educational standards through accreditation, assembles research data on employment, education, and other areas, provides consultation, develops and evaluates testing tools, and publishes a wide variety of timely books and newsletters.

The Community Health Accreditation Program (CHAP), a subsidiary of the National League for Nursing, is one of the two nationally recognized accrediting organizations for home and community health agencies. CHAP is unique because it involves patients and other users of care in the process of defining quality in community and home health care.

Its accredited agencies include clinics, community health/public health nursing centers, hospices, organizations providing professional and paraprofessional services, home medical equipment/supply companies, and agencies providing private duty nurses and supplemental staffing. These groups might offer such services as nursing, social work, physical therapy, speech therapy, occupational therapy, respiratory therapy, homemakers, home health aides, pharmacy, or nutrition counseling.

Say NLN, also referred to as "The League," and you think of education. Many nursing school faculty participate in the organization through one of its four educational membership councils:

Council of Associate Degree Programs, Council of Baccalaureate and Higher Degree Programs, Council of Diploma Programs, or the Council of Practical Nursing Programs. The councils develop criteria and guidelines for evaluating educational programs to be accredited.

Accreditation aims to maintain and enhance educational quality, thus contributing to the improvement of nursing practice. The League is recognized by the United States Department of Education as the accrediting body for nursing.

Other important services include the NLN consultation network, which provides a select group of experts in such areas as education, communication, research, and testing, who work with schools, hospitals, and health care agencies. The Division of Assessment and Evaluation runs the largest professional testing service in the country, and the Division of Research assembles highly reliable data by conducting large-scale surveys and performing detailed analysis on the entire universe of nursing education and supply. Survey response rates are as high as 90 percent.

Another popular service is the Division of Multimedia Communications which distributes a treasure trove of informative material, including publications and videos. NLN publishes an official journal, *N&HC (Nursing and Health Care): Perspectives on Community* and a membership newsletter *NLN Update*.

As the international honor society of nursing, **Sigma Theta Tau International** (STTI) selects students enrolled in NLN-accredited programs leading to a baccalaureate or higher degree. The criteria for selection includes high academic achievement, demonstration of outstanding leadership qualities, and a capacity for personal and professional growth. STTI encourages creative problem solving, cultivates high professional standards, and seeks to foster nursing's ideals.

The organization spearheaded the development of the International Center for Nursing Scholarship built in 1989. It has an ongoing fund-raising campaign for the Virginia Henderson International Nursing Library which provides a registry of nurse researchers and their projects, a research fund, and the nursing leadership institute.

In 1994, 345 chapters were active in all 50 states and Canada, Puerto Rico, Korea, Australia, and Taiwan with more than 105,000 active members. STTI's top priority is research with many chapters granting scholarships and funds for nurses engaged in studies. Its official publication and the most widely read scholarly nursing journal is the quarterly *Image: The Journal of Nursing Scholarship.*

SHARPENING YOUR PUBLISHING SKILLS

One thing most associations have in common is that they publish an official journal. Reading professional journals will keep you up-to-date on nursing issues and clinical breakthroughs. At present, these publications run the gamut from administration and education to general and advanced clinical practice. Some zero in on professional development issues, research, and especially on specialty practice which is featured in more than 50 journals.

With the many publications available, nurses are eager to publish. Who knows, you may too. You'll want to share what you're doing in your practice with other nurses and health professionals. Maybe later on when you become a seasoned writer, you will explore writing for the public. When Dorothy Brooten of the school of nursing, University of Pennsylvania, described her research, it was reported all over the country in the mass media. Her topic was on the satisfaction of patients and the safety and cost savings of the early discharge of preemies with follow-up care by a clinical nurse specialist.

Being published also helps you to become known as an expert in a particular specialty or about a timely issue or development. This visibility can lead to speaking invitations at conferences and conventions and even to writing a chapter or authoring a book on the subject. It's a terrific ego booster, and who knows, with some fame you might even earn a little fortune.

RESEARCH IMPROVES PATIENT CARE

Why care about research? Because in nursing, it will add to the body of knowledge and improve patient care. Don't be fooled into thinking that nursing research is just for "those PhD types!" Even though research is undertaken at the doctoral level, there are lots of opportunities for staff nurses to participate in research in the clinical setting.

Lauren Arnold, the clinical director, obstetrical and neonatal nursing, at Philadelphia's University of Pennsylvania Medical Center, and an associate professor at the school of nursing, is involved in investigating health service delivery issues. Her research focuses on designing systems to improve efficiency and the outcome of patient care.

"Participation in research is important," Arnold explains, "because it expands thinking and matures an individual's problem-solving approaches." She believes that staff nurses can participate through a number of avenues. For example, they can assist in collecting data as part of a larger multidisciplinary project and can help identify researchable problems. While only BSN nurses and MSN candidates or graduates are used by the research team, all staff nurses have the ability to disseminate and implement the findings of nursing research. When you are an RN, that creative curiosity and desire to know more can help you give better patient care.

* * *

As you have seen, becoming a nurse doesn't stop at graduation and getting a job. With a long and ambitious future ahead of you, you will enhance your career if you enter your profession with enthusiasm. Join and participate in organizations, read the literature, and keep up with the issues.

You'll get more out of nursing by putting more of yourself into it. Become active as a student and stay involved throughout your career.

10

Pacesetters in Nursing: Views from the Top

THE NURSE IN PROFESSIONAL ORGANIZATIONS

Your appointment has come through! The desire to switch gears from clinician, teacher, or some other job to the staff of a professional nursing association has borne fruit. For some time, you've been active as a volunteer in organizations, participating on various committees and task forces along with attending conferences and conventions. Now you want to be part of the behind-the-scene action at the headquarter's office. And why not? Such a challenge is hard to match in any other nonclinical setting.

As a staff member, you will be expected to provide the kind of experience that will test your worldly wisdom about the profession-at-large as well as your expertise in a particular area. It will take administrative know-how, good communication skills, and creative talent. Above all, you must believe in the goals of the organization and have a commitment to carry them out to the best of your ability.

The scope of your responsibilities will depend to a large extent upon the nature of the employing group, whether it operates at national, state (or regional), or local levels, and, of course, the membership composition. Nurses joining the staff of national organizations, such as the American Nurses Association, National League for Nursing, or one of the many specialty associations revel in all the activity that pervades the working environment.

Employees in professional staff positions have found that this type of position offers an opportunity hard to match in any other nonclinical setting. Their charge is to carry out policy set by the association's members through the board of directors (sometimes referred to as governing board or board of trustees). They accomplish this by collaborating with other staff, guiding volunteers in committee tasks, preparing working papers and materials for decision making, planning meetings and events, and speaking before numerous nursing and other groups.

Staff people rate job satisfaction quite high, which probably explains why they remain in organizational work for several years. It is fulfilling to have close contact with nursing leaders as well as younger nurses on the way up. Although some RNs regard their appointment as a great learning experience, they perceive it as an interim step in their career. Eventually, they return to clinical practice or the university, or become involved in some new nursing pursuit.

Here's how Patricia Moccia, the chief executive officer of the National League for Nursing, views her rise to the top of a 16 million dollar corporation that has grown in stature and resources since she assumed the helm in 1993 (see Figure 10.1). Her progression through the ranks appears to have followed a natural pattern, but she admits to no specific plan when beginning her career.

"I just wanted to learn and grow in my profession." And that she has done indeed, from staff nurse all the way up to becoming chair of the department of nursing education at Teachers College, Columbia University, a post she held for three years before coming to NLN.

A youthful, dynamic leader with boundless energy, Moccia is a person of vision who credits as her mentors the professors she had at New York University, where she earned all her academic degrees from bachelor's to PhD. "They were models of professional women who greatly influenced my life," she says, recalling with some nostalgia her student days in the 1960s and 1970s.

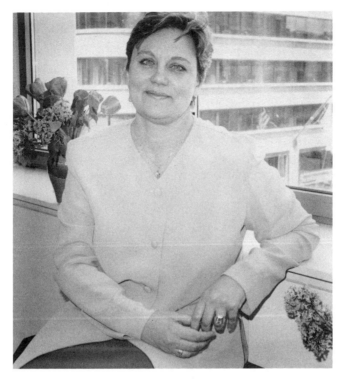

Figure 10.1 Patricia Moccia, Chief Executive Officer of the National League for Nursing.

Her prototype of an earlier vintage was the spirited nursing leader and suffragist Lavinia Dock, whom she discovered in an undergraduate history of nursing course. "When I speak before student groups, I always say that I come to them in the tradition of Miss Dock. She was a great social activist and I admire that."

You might say that Moccia's devotion to public service has almost a "genetic" basis. "My father was a fireman in Queens, New York, and very involved in the community," she explains. "Helping society is a value that I was taught by his example—to live by. And I cherish it."

What does it take to be the CEO of a prominent corporation? Moccia responds quickly. "Courage," she laughs. "Seriously, however, you need to have the physical strength and intellectual commitment to do what has to be done. More than that," she adds, "you must be able to trust people. That is, trust their potential. They need to know what you are trying to do since you can't do it all yourself."

As an executive, she believes her role is to create an environment that will bring the right people together with the right values. During her tenure, NLN has moved its programming toward a stronger community focus. "This shift is in keeping with the times. Not only have we strengthened our relationships with community groups, but our staff is increasingly interdisciplinary. We have specialists in epidemiology, primary care, public health, and other areas."

As a nursing organization, one of NLN's unique features is that its support comes from many sources. "We want to increase our non-nurse membership to help meet the overall goal of advancing the health of diverse communities through nursing."

Moccia is much in demand for speaking engagements as well as serving as a member, or in an advisory capacity, on committees and boards of health and public policy groups. Always on the go, she still manages to pursue other interests away from the organizational scene. One of her greatest pleasures comes from reading.

Any favorite topics?

She pauses a moment and smiles, "*Everything!*"

THE NURSE IN PUBLISHING

From *reading* to *writing* seems like a logical transition. At least, that's the view of editors of nursing journals and those in publishing houses, and they ought to know. Sitting behind their desks in the editorial catbird seat, they wave that wand which carries a lot of influence. So, it is fair game to characterize these nurses as pacesetters in the profession.

Someday you too may aspire to becoming a nursing editor. No, it is not an impossible dream, but first you must earn that honor and then live up to the expectations of your authors, readers, and colleagues.

Nurse editors represent a comparatively new breed. Up until two decades ago, nursing journals were few and far between. What followed was an amazing transformation with the clinical specialization movement, which led to the formation of national nursing specialty groups. Before long, a flurry of journals became visible, numbering 22 by the mid-1970s. By the early 1990s, the number of nursing journals representing various interests reached the remarkable figure of 100 or more.

Since publishing the writings of nurses is an important part of their professional development and contributes to nursing's body of knowledge, you can see why editors play such a key role. If the idea intrigues you, then you probably want to know more about this stimulating field. And who better to share these thoughts with you than a real pro like Suzanne Smith Blancett, the highly respected editorial head of the *Journal of Nursing Administration (JONA)* and *Nurse Educator*. Her story will inspire you (see Figure 10.2).

"I can't remember a moment when I didn't want to be a nurse," she says, vividly recalling all the Cherry Ames books she read while growing up in New England in the 1940s and 1950s. "I was thrilled that I might be part of such an exciting environment as the hospital and become as accomplished as my fictional heroine."

In her formative years, strong women influenced her development as well as her thinking. A grandmother, aunt, and her mother had endured the hardships of immigration, economic depression, and some tragic family events. "They gave me values of self-reliance and perseverance along with a sense of service to the community. And they emphasized the power of education and accomplishing goals through hard work."

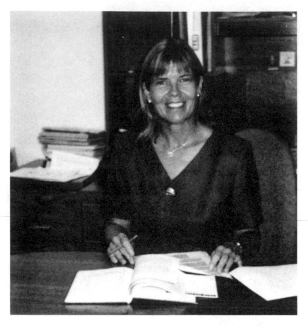

Figure 10.2 Suzanne Smith Blancett, Editor-in-Chief, *Journal of Nursing Administration* and *Nurse Educator.*

A love of English grammar and composition can be traced to her childhood when family members constantly read to her until she could make out the words herself. "When I was five years old, I got my first library card and went through just about every book in the children's section!"

Blancett's formal introduction to nursing began with her acceptance to the program at Simmons College in Boston. Following work experience in psychiatric nursing, teaching in a baccalaureate program, and then completing a master's degree in community nursing from Boston University, she returned to school to earn her doctorate. In early 1981, she planned to resume teaching when an ad in the *Boston Globe* caught her eye: *Wanted—Assistant to the Editor, Nursing Education.*

After convincing the editor and publisher that she was the person for the job, Blancett joined the staff of *Nurse Educator*. "Being a fast learner, I quickly caught on though I knew next to nothing," she declares. "However, with a good grasp of English and reading hundreds of manuscripts, I soon was editing for clarity."

She claims that her nursing education background provided the basic skills to be a successful editor. "I knew how to deal with people and how to teach and set goals. I also had learned how to assess, plan, and evaluate the work at hand, think critically, and do some problem solving."

Within two years, a promotion to director of the editorial and marketing department took Blancett into the realm of production, circulation, and other areas. In the 1980s, when the J.B. Lippincott Company purchased *Nurse Educator* and another magazine called *JONA,* she was appointed editor-in-chief of the two publications. Her responsibilities enlarged considerably but she was well able to handle them assisted by her staff. At that time, she also had family responsibilities raising a teenage son and daughter.

What does she find most satisfying about her job? "Just what I like about nursing—working with people. As an editor, I am able to help writers achieve their goal of getting their ideas disseminated. I have great respect for the time and effort they put into their work."

Her job requires several skills, such as knowing the needs of the readers of both journals, and being aware of trends and issues in health as they concern nurse administrators and educators. Assisting her in manuscript review is a team of expert editorial advisors whom she selects carefully.

Does she have some words of wisdom for prospective nurse editors? "Get experience and get involved in the process. Do articles for your agency newsletter and then start writing for your specialty journal." When nurses attend conferences or conventions, she urges them to seek out the exhibit booths of publishers. "Introduce yourself to journal and book editors and share your ideas."

Although Blancett misses clinical practice, she still considers herself a teacher bringing knowledge about the field to her readers. "I take my role seriously as a gatekeeper of information. And

I appreciate the opportunity to meet and know the best and the brightest in nursing."

NURSE ENTREPRENEURS: AS THE SPIRIT MOVES

You now have some familiarity with nursing jobs in nonclinical areas, just as you have learned in earlier chapters from nurses first-hand about practice in hospitals and in the community. Other RNs, however, have bitten the proverbial bullet and decided to strike out on their own. Some have established independent companies or agencies, either alone or with a partner or two, and in all cases they continue to use their nursing knowledge and skills. You would probably be surprised to know that over 20,000 nurses have their own businesses and the number is on the rise.

Perhaps you think of the entrepreneurial spirit in nursing as a new phenomenon, but this is not the case. For the moment, recall the private duty nurse, who as far back as the turn of the century considered herself an independent contractor. Private duty nurses, however, weren't the only ones.

Here's an amusing little tale and a true one right out of the nursing annals of the early 1900s. It appears that a "tired, trained nurse," who had reached the ripe old age of 34 or 35, decided to seek new directions in her profession. So, this resourceful woman contacted a physician colleague and asked him to refer his patients requiring shampoos and hair care. Before long, she became quite proficient and well-known in her specialty, one that she called *Nursing the Hair!*

Although nurse entrepreneurs in the 1990s may be involved in far more complicated enterprises than our nurse above, most seem to have that same pioneering drive, desire, and determination. You may wonder what makes a person want to chance an uncertain future and leave the security of a potentially long-term job with a stable employer and steady income. Yet, those nurses who have taken the plunge share a common belief. The most compelling reason, they say, is the need to create or try something new while contributing their nursing expertise.

120

The idea of starting a business may be an exciting prospect but it can conjure up some scary thoughts. There's always that fear of the unknown. At the same time, to begin such an adventure (which it truly is) means that you have to be a risk taker. And as you know, risks may involve pain but they can also bring great pleasure. By accentuating the positive, your hopes for a bright business future are far more promising.

In many cases, remarkable successes have followed with nurses developing lucrative businesses around the country. A number of entrepreneurs are nurse practitioners and clinical specialists sharing private practices. In addition, there are RNs, including a number of male nurses, who previously held administrative positions in hospitals, nursing schools, and other agencies.

Some of the services offered are women's health and wellness, home health care, mammography programs in nurse-managed centers, dialysis care, CPR (cardiopulmonary resuscitation) classes, and medical/legal consultation. Also, independently run nursing firms perform executive searches or operate registries for supplying staff in homes and hospitals. Another popular venture is forming a company sponsoring continuing education workshops and conferences on clinical and educational topics.

Caroline Camuñas has maintained an unusually active life-style since 1990 when she and two other nurse colleagues opened Nurse Executive Associates, Inc. in New York City. As consultants, they offer expert guidance in nursing service administration. All three were seasoned administrators as well as educators who had been involved in individual consultation.

The notion of a combined undertaking first came about when Camuñas and fellow faculty member Ruth Alward were collaborating on a book about marketing for professional nurses. At the time, they decided that it might not be a bad idea to "market themselves," and before long, with the addition of Judy Cassells, they were in business.

Although Camuñas continues to provide some consultation in administration, her changing goals have taken her in another direction. A long time interest as well as study in the area of nursing ethics has prepared her to meet a growing need in the nursing community. Ethical concerns in patient care have become more visible with different health problems, more technology, and people wanting information about their condition and care. (See *Code of Ethics for Nurses,* p. 147.)

"We talk about family values today and that has a great deal to do with ethics in general," she says. "In health care there have been many ethical issues, such as confidentiality, informed consent, and the patient's right to make decisions about his own care. Our job as nurses is to give the person support and guidance and then assist him in deciding what to do."

Camuñas admits that although her work is challenging, there are no easy answers. "For example, when a patient has an infectious disease and refuses treatment, he not only harms himself but he may expose others to the infection. So, the nurse has to work with him in solving the problem."

And how is that done?

"By listening and by asking the right questions if the patient is to get the right information," she explains.

As a consultant, Camuñas meets with many groups and individuals—nurses, hospital residents, patients in rehabilitation centers and other settings, and families of patients. She confers with physicians, psychologists, and numerous health professionals.

Becoming an ethicist, she explains, requires a broad-based educational background that includes not only the scientific basis of nursing but a strong foundation in the humanities. "After all, nursing is a highly humanistic profession."

Always eager to learn more about her specialty, she spent a year, beginning in June 1994, as a fellow at the Joseph and Rose Kennedy Institute of Ethics, Georgetown University in Washington, DC. There, she expanded her knowledge of ethics in general, participating in discussions about health care reform, genetics, and reproductive technology. A high point of the experience was working with the institute's senior research scholars, Edmund Pellegrino, a physician and medical ethicist, and the philosopher Thomas Beachchamp.

Camuñas notes that she isn't the only busy professional in her family. She and her husband, a cardio-thoracic surgeon, manage to relax by going to their country house in upstate New York, close to where she grew up. "We love it there and I get a chance to do my gardening," she laughs. "I guess you could say that I literally have gone back to my roots!"

Professional nurse consultants encompass all areas of nursing. They operate in many different ways with some self-employed like Caroline Camuñas, or a nurse attorney in private practice called upon to consult on legal/health issues. A number of faculty members and nurse administrators in health care institutions also do consultation apart from their primary position. A number of local, state, national, and international organizations, both private and public, employ consultants. You will find consultants working with major foundations, serving as lobbyists, labor relations specialists, or liaisons to pharmaceutical companies and other groups.

* * *

Many options exist for professional nurses who continue to contribute to improving patient care and the quality of life. While some practice at the bedside, others reach out to nonclinical settings where their impact may be just as great in a less direct fashion. The attractiveness of self-employment and having special services to offer is gaining momentum in the profession. You too may want to pursue this route in time. Certainly, career mobility has a magic ring in the nursing marketplace!

11

The Wide World of Nursing

Wherever you find people in need, you'll find nurses. Around the world or around the corner, nurses are there. And often they find themselves in the most unexpected situations. Take, for example, what happened to Keith Bradkowski, on the morning of January 17, 1994. His compelling story shows the actions of nurses and their commitment to patients.

In California people expect and respect earthquakes. No one, including Bradkowski, was quite prepared for what many thought was "the big one." The administrative director, patient care services, at Santa Monica-UCLA Medical Center, was jolted out of bed at 4:32 A.M. Bradkowski jumped into his car and headed for his hospital.

He arrived to discover that the emergency electrical backup system had failed. His first concern: the patients on ventilators. Rushing through the hospital with water gushing from ceilings made him feel like he was living in a disaster movie. Aftershocks rocked the building, often knocking down ceiling tiles and springing new water leaks.

In the critical care unit, he found the nurses standing beside their patients in total darkness. Two patients dependent on ventilators were breathing just fine. The staff had been artificially ventilating them since the power went out over an hour before. The hospital emergency incident command system was working. Only a month before the earthquake, the hospital had a disaster drill and everyone was well prepared. But there were other serious problems.

One of the hospital's two buildings had been declared unsafe. All patients and staff had to be moved to the newer pavilion. To make matters worse, Saint John's Hospital, three blocks away, was being closed entirely due to damage. "Our facility was the only health care institution in the Santa Monica area," Bradkowski relates. Patients were rushing into the emergency room with injuries.

Throughout the hours and days after the quake, the staff and community rallied together. Nurses and physicians from the area appeared at the hospital to volunteer their services. The skilled nursing facility was closed and patients were moved to other locations. Within two days, everything had been reorganized into one very crowded building. The medical center was in "disaster mode" for the next two months. Bradkowski said that he saw firsthand that "heroes are those who do the best of things during the worst of times." Santa Monica's health care professionals proved it.

So did the health care professionals in Oklahoma City, OK. When a terrorist bomb rocked Oklahoma City and the entire country on April 19, 1995, nurses rushed to help. Calls from around the country swamped the phones at the Oklahoma Nurses Association offering to assist in any way they could. In less than ten hours, one thousand calls were logged from RNs, LPNs, nurses' aides, and physicians.

Fortunately, the city and state's health care personnel came together in support. Less than two hours after the blast, all kinds of health professionals were on the scene to help the victims. With compassion, these nurses and others cared for people with terrible injuries. In the aftermath of the disaster, psychiatric nurses have continued to counsel the affected families and also their health care colleagues to cope with the emotions of the ordeal.

RED CROSS NURSING

Red Cross nurses rally in the worst of times. When floods devastated the Midwest in 1993, they were there working long hours as members of the disaster teams. RNs worked as educators, medics, and health care consultants. That rescue effort alone cost more than $30 million, the third most expensive effort in Red Cross history. Annually, the American Red Cross deals with close to 60,000 natural and manmade disasters through its local chapters. A private agency, it survives mainly on the generous support of the people it serves.

Clara Barton founded the American Red Cross in 1881. This humanitarian volunteer organization provides direct relief to victims of disasters and helps communities prepare for and respond to emergencies. It is also well-known for its efforts to maintain the country's blood supply through donations. In addition, Red Cross nurses serve as instructors in educational programs for the public on subjects from first aid and CPR, to babysitting and parenting. Another important role of the Red Cross is providing emergency communications, financial help, and counseling services to the families of service men and women during war and peacetime on United States military bases worldwide.

On the international scene, the organization is at the forefront of humanitarian relief efforts at sites of natural disasters and, all too often, in war zones. It helps to locate and reunite those separated from their families. Red Cross nurses in paid and volunteer roles are a valuable resource, helping communities meet their health care needs. You can find these and other nursing heroes everywhere, just doing their jobs.

UNITED STATES PUBLIC HEALTH SERVICE

From high-tech hospitals to rustic settings in Appalachian hollows, nurses in the United States Public Health Service (PHS) work in every imaginable nursing specialty. The PHS comes under the Department of Health and Human Services and is the governmental agency responsible for overseeing the nation's health. You've probably heard of most of its eight agencies: the Food and Drug Administration, the National Institutes of Health and Substance Abuse, Indian Health Service, Centers for Disease Control and Prevention, Agency for Health Care Policy and Research, Health Resources Services Administration, Mental Health Service Administration, and the Agency for Toxic Substances and Disease Registry.

The majority of clinical opportunities can be found in the Indian Health Service (IHS) and the National Institutes of Health (NIH). Close to half of the 5,000 RNs in the PHS are employed by the IHS working in health care facilities mostly in the West. Another 800 nurses work for the NIH Clinical Center in Bethesda, MD.

A nurse can enter the PHS from two routes: the Commissioned Corps and civil service. A baccalaureate from an NLN-accredited college or university is required for entry into the Commissioned Corps. In addition, applicants must be no older than 44 years of age, be United States citizens, be licensed as RNs, and meet certain required health and physical standards. Although Corps officers can also be assigned to the Coast Guard, Federal Bureau of Prisons, Health Care Financing Administration, Immigration and Naturalization Service, and the National Oceanic and Atmospheric Administration, opportunities are more limited than for the IHS and NIH.

The Commissioned Corps is an all-officer corps of health care professionals and makes up one of the nation's seven uniformed services. The President can declare the PHS a military service in the event of war or national emergency. Commissioned Corps nurses enjoy a range of excellent benefits such as use of commissary and other base facilities, and 30 days' annual leave beginning with the first year of service. While the members have a choice of practice site, they are subject to relocation.

RNs entering the civil service can be graduates of associate degree, hospital diploma, or baccalaureate nursing programs. Grade and salary are determined by the education and experience required of the position. These nurses receive pay and benefits comparable to those of commissioned nurses, including overtime, premium pay for work on Sundays and holidays, and paid moving expenses as required.

128

THE INDIAN HEALTH SERVICE

Leslie Dye, an Indian Health Service nurse recruiter covering the Portland and Albuquerque areas, has been with the agency most of his professional life. Ask this 1979 graduate of the University of Oklahoma why working in the IHS is rewarding and he'll tell you without hesitation, "It's the people we serve. That's what it's all about." It's refreshing to work with people of different cultures, he explains, especially the graciousness of the Indian and Alaskan natives. "They really appreciate what you're doing for them."

Dye believes that the IHS provides an enjoyable working environment for nurses, who really have a chance to use their skills. "Functioning as generalists, you can use what you learned," he emphasizes. "And the physicians and other health care team members have a truly humanitarian view of why they went into medicine and health."

RNs work either for the IHS or for one of the tribes. Those hired by tribally-operated facilities are called "direct hires," while nurses working in IHS clinics, Indian hospitals and medical centers, and public outreach programs are federal employees. The latter can select from three distinct practice areas. *Hospital-based nursing practice* is for nurse generalists and nurses with specialties in OR, obstetrics, pediatrics, ICU, and emergency room. *Ambulatory care nurse practice* places nurses in the hospital setting as well as in free-standing IHS health centers. Lastly, IHS *public health nursing practice* emphasizes patient care and the assessment of community needs and focuses primarily on maternal and child care. Applicants must have a BSN and at least one year's experience.

Advanced practice nurses can find considerable autonomy within the IHS where a great need exists for nurse practitioners, certified nurse-midwives, and certified registered nurse anesthetists. A federal employment option enables APNs to practice, subject only to the limitations of their original state license, no matter where their IHS facility is located.

Sound too good to be true? Well, there's more. The IHS also offers educational loan repayment of up to $25,000 per year toward the principal, interest, and related expenses on government and commercial loans for nursing education. Reimbursable costs include tuition, books, and reasonable living expenses. In exchange, nurses serve for at least two years at an IHS facility.

THE NIH CLINICAL CENTER

The National Institutes of Health in Bethesda, MD, is the world center for research. Located on the 360-acre NIH campus, the Clinical Center is the largest hospital in the world dedicated entirely to biomedical research. It houses 450 patient beds and employs more than 800 nurses.

There are slots for new graduates as well as experienced nurses. In fact, the Center provides a comprehensive, unit-based preceptorship for all new nurses (see Figure 11.1). In addition, many areas of specialization offer their own intensive training and internship programs. NIH has a low patient-to-nurse ratio allowing the staff to practice primary nursing on a highly individualized basis. Patients

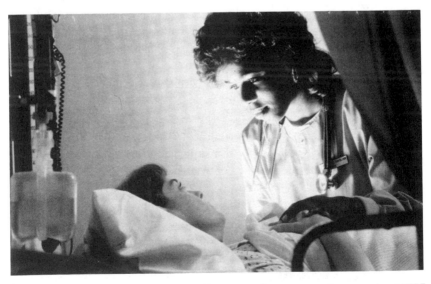

Figure 11.1   Janice Adams offers support to a patient at the NIH Clinical Center in Bethesda, MD.

are referred by physicians worldwide. Nurses may choose from more than 50 clinics and nursing units from geriatrics to pediatrics, ambulatory care to intensive care, and chronic care to acute care.

The stimulating educational environment fosters opportunities to attend courses and seminars, nursing grand rounds, conferences, conventions, and clinical inservices, attractive perks including competitive salary, tuition assistance and clinical ladder for advancement, child care, relocation expenses, paid holidays and sick leave, and up to 26 vacation days.

THE NATIONAL HEALTH SERVICE CORPS AND COSTEP

Two special PHS programs also exist. The National Health Service Corps, established in 1970, recruits health care professionals for underserved areas. In exchange for financial assistance, participants agree to a minimum of two years' service in urban and rural communities. Primary care nurse practitioners and certified nurse midwives are the nursing specialties most in demand.

Competition is keen but junior students in BSN programs can apply for COSTEP, the Commissioned Officer Student Training and Extern Program and Senior COSTEP program. They receive clinical assignments from one to four months' duration in PHS agencies across the country. You can earn more than $1,900 a month while gaining experience and insight into public health activities. Unfortunately, budget restraints affect opportunities in both the National Health Service Corps and the COSTEP programs.

DEPARTMENT OF VETERANS AFFAIRS HEALTH CARE FACILITIES

Another opportunity in the federal government is in the VA system which operates over 170 hospitals and 200 clinics ranging in size from 100 to more than 1,400 beds and employs more than

35,000 RNs. As the country's largest health care provider, the VA runs national programs that aid and care for the veterans of the armed forces. Many of the hospitals are teaching facilities affiliated with schools of medicine, nursing, and related health care professions.

The VA provides a broad range of care for medical, surgical, psychiatric, and nursing home patients as well as specialty care in programs such as critical care, substance abuse treatment, hemodialysis, spinal cord injury, organ transplant, and ambulatory care. Graduates of all nursing programs may apply. Applicants must be United States citizens and meet certain required physical standards. New graduates are accepted for employment pending licensure.

NURSING IN THE MILITARY

Nurses in the military have a unique opportunity not just to practice nursing but to experience the world, and maybe even make history at the same time. Talk to them and you will find a high level of excitement and satisfaction about their work, their educational opportunities for growth, the working environment, and other benefits. One military nurse says her life took a new direction as soon as she reached her first assignment. Not only did she meet lifelong friends (including her husband), but she was thrilled to have an opportunity to refine her clinical and management skills. After her first duty station, she made the Army her full-time career.

All branches of the military emphasize continuing education, and usually fund, at least partially, master's education for advanced practice. RNs enjoy many fringe benefits such as high quality medical and dental care, housing allowances, low cost life insurance, generous paid vacations, and excellent retirement benefits. And, of course, there's always the opportunity to travel, while stationed at military facilities around the nation and the world.

A special feeling of camaraderie among colleagues goes unmatched in the armed services. "You're part of a team, a family," one nurse commented. "Wherever you go in the world, you can run into an old friend."

The Army Nurse Corps, Navy Nurse Corps, and Air Force Nurse Corps represent separate and distinct entities. While there are differences, a number of similarities exist, such as entering the service as a commissioned officer. In the Army Nurse Corps, an RN will normally be commissioned as a second lieutenant and can advance to the rank of brigadier general. In the Navy, appointments depend on education and other qualifications, and range from ensign to lieutenant. Navy nurses can rise through the ranks to the office of rear admiral. Air Force nurses are usually commissioned as second lieutenants and can reach the rank of brigadier general.

Each branch of service consists of a reserve corps which provides a bank of practitioners from which to draw in the event of war or national emergency. In fact, more than 75 percent of the medical strength of the military is in the reserves. If you meet the requirements, which are similar to the regular service, you'll receive training and be expected to give usually one weekend per month and two weeks consecutively at a military health care facility on an annual basis.

ARMY NURSE CORPS

Army Nurse Corps (ANC) is the oldest service, tracing its roots to 1901. Army nurses might serve anywhere in the United States or throughout the world. You'll find them delivering direct patient care, serving as teachers, doing research, advising nurses from other nations, and much much more.

Whether on active duty or in the reserve, Army nurses combine a military career with clinical practice. Ronalda Futtrell-Hobson was recently promoted to the rank of colonel after 16 years in the Army Nurse Corps, United States Army Reserve. Futtrell-Hobson, a family nurse practitioner (FNP) and certified sex therapist was selected over 739 lieutenant colonels who qualified for promotion in 1993.

As a FNP at the Family Medicine Office, St. Anthony's Hospital at Sanderlin, FL, she and her colleagues provide primary health care to entire families, particularly women and children.

"I see patients, make referrals, write prescriptions, and especially love the health teaching," she says.

During Operation Desert Shield/Desert Storm in 1991, she was called up to active duty. In her first assignment, she assisted the Preventive Medicine-Community Health Nursing Operation at Lyster Army Hospital, Ft. Rucker, Alabama. At the beginning of Desert Storm, she was ordered to Fitzsimmons Army Medical Center, Colorado, to help in the expansion of the medical center to receive anticipated casualties arriving from Saudi Arabia. Fortunately, casualties were almost nonexistent and Futtrell-Hobson returned to Ft. Rucker as demobilization officer to direct a team providing epidemiological and public health care to 5,000 returning soldiers. "We interviewed every returning GI and listened to them share their physical and emotional concerns," she explains.

According to Futtrell-Hobson, military nursing is special because of the opportunity to develop leadership skills. "You're working as an officer, side by side with those in combat and combat-support roles. There's an amazing opportunity to hone your own skills while developing and challenging others. You're always stretching."

Her current military assignment is as the United States Military Academy Liaison Officer for the Southeast region where she is responsible for marketing and recruiting activities. She interviews prospective West Point candidates and frequently meets with guidance counselors and legislators regarding Academy appointees. In the event of a mobilization, she would serve as the Chief, Nursing Administrator, at Ft. Meade, Maryland.

Nurses interested in joining the ANC must be graduates of an accredited program preparing for RN licensure. Those seeking active duty must have a baccalaureate in nursing or nurse anesthesia. Applicants for reserve status can be graduates from associate degree, hospital diploma, or baccalaureate degree nursing programs; hold licensure as a registered nurse; be between the ages of 21 and 48 and be United States citizens; have worked at least six months as an RN for no less than 20 hours per week in the year prior to applying for service; and be capable of meeting the physical standards of military service. Applicants may be single or married with dependents of any age.

134

NAVY NURSE CORPS

If you like the water, nurses should consider the Navy Nurse Corps (NNC). You'll find navy nurses on ships and in duty stations around the world. They provide direct patient care in a wide variety of clinical specialties as well as serve as teachers, researchers, administrators, and in other capacities.

Applicants must meet the following requirements: be a graduate of an accredited program preparing for licensure as a registered nurse. Those seeking active duty must hold a baccalaureate or an advanced degree or an associate degree or a diploma from a hospital school with no less than 108 academic weeks *and* a baccalaureate degree in a related field, such as chemistry, biology, psychology, or health sciences; be a U.S. citizen; licensed as an RN and certified if a nurse anesthetist or nurse practitioner; be of strong moral character; be actively involved in nursing practice with excellent references; and have the physical stamina required by the Navy. RNs must be able to serve 20 years of active duty before reaching the age of 55. (Some exceptions are made in certain nursing specialties.) NNC applicants may be married or single.

AIR FORCE NURSE CORPS

The dream of being a flight nurse might attract you to the Air Force Nurse Corps (AFNC). The majority of air force nurses, however, work on land in hospitals, medical centers, and clinics in the United States and abroad. They serve as nurse anesthetists, in operating rooms, as nurse practitioners, and certified nurse midwives, to name a few specialties.

To be a flight nurse involved in aeromedical activities, you must first complete a comprehensive educational program preparing you to manage and treat patients in flight. Nurses study techniques for proper transfer of patients, aerospace physiology, and survival principles.

Applicants for the Air Force Nurse Corps must be U.S. citizens, at least 18 years of age, able to meet physical standards, and be graduates of a nursing school recognized by the Surgeon General of

135

the Air Force. They must also be licensed as registered nurses, can be married or single, and have dependents of any age.

OPPORTUNITIES OVERSEAS

Nursing is a career packed with opportunities for international travel. As a nurse, you can work and experience the world at the same time. There are a number of agencies, other than the military, which offer creative challenges and the experience of working in a foreign country.

THE PEACE CORPS

Peace Corps nurses in Paraguay provide clinical and teaching assistance by developing health education programs through community health facilities and schools. In Malawi, public health nurses work in rural clinics working to improve sanitation and health care practices, and in Zaire, they work in cooperation with the World Health Organization, USAID, and other international agencies in a child survival program.

Nurses can discover a wide range of experiences in any of the 60 Peace Corps countries around the world. Regardless of their assigned site, volunteers work with host country nurses and health workers within the framework of existing health services. The volunteer's primary function will be the training of other nurses and health personnel, always emphasizing the involvement of the community and its own health needs.

RNs from all nursing programs can qualify, although education and experience in public health nursing are valuable. Before starting a two-year assignment, volunteers receive cross-cultural and language instruction and locale-specific technical training as needed. The role of a Peace Corps volunteer or staff nurse isn't for everyone. If you are flexible, patient, independent, and don't mind working and living in what might be spartan conditions, the assignment can be a rewarding highlight of your career.

136

WORLD HEALTH ORGANIZATION

As with the Peace Corps, the World Health Organization (WHO) employs nurses with advanced clinical skills and language skills for international assignments. One of the largest agencies of the United Nations, WHO assists governments around the world on request with their health problems. The agency also provides health programs in individual countries, particularly in the improvement of health care for women and babies. WHO nurses serve in advisory roles to aid local nurses with particular health concerns, although they sometimes must provide direct care until one of the nurses in the community acquires the education and training to assume the task.

WHO seeks highly skilled RNs with expertise in a needed area. Its official languages are English, Spanish, French, Russian, Arabic, and Chinese. WHO nurses must be fluent in at least one language other than their own.

AGENCY FOR INTERNATIONAL DEVELOPMENT

The Agency for International Development (AID) is administered by the United States Department of State, although its activities take place worldwide. AID hires a limited number of RNs to accomplish short or long-term projects. Like WHO, the organization assists nations in such areas as public health nursing, midwifery services, education of ancillary health workers, and establishing nursing education programs, especially at postgraduate levels preparing nurses for teaching and administration. At present, AID funds a limited number of nursing activities.

PROJECT HOPE

Project Hope, on the other hand, has an active nursing component although it is targeted primarily to RNs with advanced education and experience. The goal of the private foundation is to "go only where invited and help others to help themselves by educating them to teach and treat their own people." While providing some limited direct care, Project Hope's activities stress the training of local individuals and developing of local health institutions. "Our saying is 'We don't give people fish, we teach them to fish,'" says Patricia Lybarger, a Project Hope volunteer since 1982.

The staff development coordinator at the Burns Institute, Boston Shriners Hospital for Crippled Children, Lybarger is at present part of an ongoing project with Children's Hospital #9 in Moscow. She is the nurse educator on a team of four health professionals charged with helping the hospital establish a multidisciplinary burn unit.

When explosions from a train wreck in the Ural Mountains in the summer of 1989 killed and severely burned many families on summer holiday, the Russian government asked the United States for help. "A number of burn teams from the military and civilian sector responded immediately, including those from several Shriners Hospitals. Later in the fall, the State Department asked Project Hope to help establish the All Union Pediatric Burn Unit at Hospital #9, and I was approached by a physician on the Project Hope team," she explains.

Lybarger had participated earlier with Project Hope helping to establish a burn unit at the university hospital in Jamaica, so she jumped at the chance to work on the Russian project. "The experience has been incredible, a little scary but exciting," she recounts, "and the project has been renewed for another five years."

"Project Hope is perfect for experienced skilled nurses who are adventurous," she points out. "But it's not for beginning your career." RNs accepted for international assignments must, at the very least, have at least two full years of work experience and be graduates of an NLN-accredited BSN program. Because of Project Hope's educational focus, students are often required to have a master's degree and academic or clinical teaching experience.

In addition to short-term volunteer experiences, Project Hope also employs full-time nurses for most projects. RNs receive salaries comparable to those in the marketplace, plus transportation and expenses for the candidate and family. Additional benefits include generous insurance plans, including life, health, and malpractice, and a retirement plan.

Some limited internship experiences are also available for those interested in a career in international health care. Interns are subjected to a competitive selection process that looks at educational preparation, skills, interests, and the student's ability to have an impact in the field. Designed with the support of the student's school, these internships vary in length. No scholarships or loan forgiveness programs currently exist.

MISSIONARY NURSING

Have you ever seen yourself as Helen Bresslau, the nurse and wife of Albert Schweitzer, who journeyed to Africa in the early 1900s with a team of medical missionaries? Schweitzer wrote: "She looked after the severe cases, superintended the linen and the bandages, was often busy in the dispensary, kept the instruments in proper condition, made all the preparations for the operations herself, then administered the anesthetics."

Some religious groups still operate missions and hospitals employing nurses. For those who want to share their religious beliefs as well as practice nursing, missionary nursing can be a satisfying career. Since church missions are often based in developing countries, nurses considering missionary nursing should be familiar with different cultures and languages other than English. Check with your religious affiliation to determine availabilities and requirements.

* * *

Where in the world do you see yourself practicing? Stimulating challenges await the nurse who seeks out nontraditional practice areas.

Whether you choose service in the military or in the United States Public Health Service, or work as a staff nurse or volunteer in the American Red Cross, your work may take you to exotic, even dangerous, locations. If you are fluent in a language other than your own, you can set your sights on jobs far and wide. For the qualified person, organizations like the Peace Corps, World Health Organization, Project Hope, and the Agency for International Development can provide unequaled experiences around the globe.

Where do you see yourself practicing? The wide world of nursing is out there waiting for you.

12

New Directions:
Greeting the Next Century

Your long day's journey into the world of professional nursing, as travelled through the pages of this book, is coming to an end. But the big adventure lies just ahead if you are sufficiently convinced— and maybe somewhat titillated—by the prospect of nursing as the career for you. Even if you knew something about the field before, you now have a lot more information at your fingertips.

You also have learned that nothing can match the joy of being directly part of the action. The firsthand vignettes shared by nurses themselves not only show the vast array of job opportunities available, but also how fulfilled nurses are in their work. Here you could capture the real excitement—a far cry from the frenetic, fictionalized arena of television drama.

THE PRESENT PICTURE

Perhaps "change" is the best way to describe nursing today. That's not surprising, of course, with all the remarkable developments occurring around the globe. Just think how dynamic the whole health field has become in the United States over the past few decades. The good news is that people live longer as a result of earlier diagnosis and treatment, healthier life-styles, self-care programs, and a greater exposure to health information. Also, death from heart disease is down due to surgical intervention and new drugs, as well as consumer awareness of better nutrition, exercise, and cessation of cigarette smoking.

The entire health care picture, however, is not all positive. On the increase are such serious problems as auto accidents, homicides, substance abuse, mental depression and anxiety disorders, and adolescent sexuality. The pregnancy of teenagers, ages 15 to 19, has created birthrates higher in our nation than those in most developed countries. Cancer, particularly of the lungs, continues to be a leading cause of death, although important strides have been made in prevention and treatment.

As you know, the most devastating as well as perplexing illness of the 1980s and 1990s is HIV and AIDS, currently reaching epidemic proportions. Another public threat, linked to AIDS, the homeless, and the drug abuser, is the reemergence of tuberculosis. These concerns and others create enormous challenges for the health professions. In time, however, scientific and medical advances will eradicate many of the present ills. Yet, new problems will inevitably appear on the horizon.

PREDICTIONS AND POSSIBILITIES

Although predictions may be risky, it is important for you to have some expectations for the future of health care. Already in evidence is a growing aging population, which by the year 2000 will consist of over 36 million Americans 65 or older, with almost half aged 75 or more. It is anticipated that many older people will be well and active much longer as medical advances reduce illness and disability. The poet, Robert Browning, may have been right on target when he said: "Grow old with me! The best is yet to be."

Medical science will open the way to new frontiers in preventing and treating genetic diseases. More curative treatments will be discovered as research continues to explore the basic causes of cancer and heart disease. In the realm of surgical transplantation, quite common at present, operations will expand in number and type, and artificial implants will increase.

Some experts predict that certain surgical procedures will decline and be replaced by lasers and advances in radiation and drug therapy. One area that scientists still ponder is the human brain and how to successfully unlock the mysteries behind such mental disorders as depression, schizophrenia, senility, and even criminal behavior. The answers, many believe, will come with the revolution in drug treatment.

A few years ago, the U.S. Public Health Service proposed several national goals in its report, *Healthy People 2000: National Health Promotion and Disease Prevention Objectives* (1991). Some of the broader areas identified related to reducing infant mortality and disability from chronic conditions, and increasing life expectancy. Also recommended was decreasing the disparity in life expectancy between white and minority populations.

There is no question about the significant role expected of technology in future health care. It may seem a bit farfetched, but with advances in artificial intelligence and computerization, patients may soon be able to obtain their diagnosis electronically at home.

The present use of computers has already had a marked impact on organizational structures like hospitals. All kinds of management information systems have been implemented in record keeping, billing, research, diagnostic application, and nursing documentation. Nurses have a pivotal role in these systems and therefore must learn as much as they can about computers.

Their involvement is crucial in planning, designing, standardizing, and evaluating the nursing database. Through nursing information systems, they can improve both cost effectiveness and the quality of patient care. In many undergraduate programs, nursing informatics courses have been introduced and, in some cases, are required.

NURSING'S CRYSTAL BALL

While preparing for nursing's future may stimulate one's imagination, it is no easy task when you consider all the present concerns. When planned, change can be advantageous since it represents a departure from the status quo. As professionals, nurses have a responsibility to advance with the times, recognizing the health care needs created by social, economic, and political forces as well as by developments in science.

Nursing practice must also change along with the organizational structures that support it. These developments will have to be incorporated into the educational system since the role of nurses will continue to evolve as well as expand. The window of opportunity in nursing's numerous employment settings will be open to those who are prepared and eager to make their contribution.

What then will be in store for you as you embark upon a career in nursing? The best part is that the projected demand will increase and, by the turn of the century, 500,000 more positions will be available to nurses. Hospitals will continue to focus increasingly on acute care and critical care for inpatients. On the other hand, ambulatory care in outpatient areas is expected to flourish.

According to the Division of Nursing, U.S. Public Health Service, 140,000 full-time registered nurses with graduate degrees (master's and doctoral) will be in the work force by the year 2000. And just think, the demand for nurses at these levels will soar. Included are RNs in teaching, research, and advanced practice, such as nurse practitioners, clinical specialists, certified nurse-midwives, and certified nurse anesthetists. Nursing organizations and many health care employers have been urging wider use of advanced practice nurses.

In earlier chapters of the book, you were alerted to the movement underway toward nursing in the community. With the early discharge of patients from hospitals—a trend expected to continue—nurses will have to intensify their services in home care. They also will be needed to provide primary care in schools, shelters, long-term care facilities, neighborhood clinics, community nursing centers, and many other sites.

The kinds of health problems facing patients in the future, and the changing nature of the population in American health care will profoundly affect the services to be rendered. Changes in the ethnicity of the consumer will require new understanding of health care practices.

144

The influx of immigrants from other lands creates fresh challenges for nurses who will be providing care to persons from multicultural and multiracial groups with differing values, interests, and language. Unlike the great European migration to the United States in the first decade of the century, the new immigrants are primarily Hispanic (from the Americas), and Asian (mainly Korean and Filipino).

Educational institutions must keep pace with these developments. An expanded range of competencies and a broad knowledge base will be expected of nurses as science expands and the health care environment changes and becomes more technological. The growth of schools of nursing located in university health science centers is a positive move toward ensuring greater communication between health professional students and faculty.

As the nation explores health care reform, the idea of prevention in health care is gaining greater momentum. Many of the most serious disorders found in clinical practice can be prevented. Wherever nurses practice, they have an opportunity to deliver preventive services, which is an important part of their independent role.

Encouraging immunizations, healthier life-styles, and early detection or screening are crucial. Remember Chris Davitt, the geriatric nurse practitioner from New Jersey, who commented on the 100 plus blood pressures done in one day at a health fair? That's what you call *prevention!* Above all, every nurse knows that the very essence of nursing is to promote health.

THE LIVING LEGENDS

Throughout its history, the profession has spawned some extraordinary nurses whose innovations have left a marked impact on the larger society. Today, nursing proudly honors those who have become living legends through their charismatic leadership and vision. To name a few, you will want to learn more about the work of such "greats" as Loretta Ford, architect of the nurse practitioner movement; M. Elizabeth Carnegie, historian and chronicler of black nurses worldwide; educator Luther Christman, who created an outstanding center of excellence in nursing;

and certified nurse-midwife Ruth Lubic, founder and director of the first childbearing center in the nation.

These nursing leaders share many commonalities, none the least being the tremendous obstacles they had to overcome in achieving their goals. The opposition they endured had not come entirely from outside the profession, since the rank and file all too often resisted internal change. As risk takers and role breakers, like the Sangers and Walds of the past, these modern day nurses ploughed unchartered territory to win over their cause. What did it take? Courage, perseverance, creativity, and a firm belief in what they were trying to do.

Nursing has other movers and shakers who come from all levels of the profession. You've met some of them already, including staff nurses, clinicians, nurse executives, entrepreneurs, and others. Each one, in their own way is making a significant difference in the lives of people.

NURSING: YOUR CAREER
OF A LIFETIME

Whether to enter the nursing profession may be one of the most important decisions that you will ever have to make. You will need to consider your choice as an investment in the future that will enrich you in many ways. Just as the field continues to grow, you too can expand your vistas to reach the heights to which you aspire. There is no limit on the hopes, dreams, and ambitions of the individual who seeks professional self-fulfillment.

As you have discovered, nursing cannot be viewed merely as one career. Rather, it is a career within a career and that is what makes it so unique—a bevy of options, a number of settings. Your professional world will never be dull because goals can change and new directions may be sought. And throughout the experience you will develop as a person in your own right.

If nursing is your choice, then go for it. Make it your career of a lifetime!

Appendix

A Code of Ethics for Nurses

The nurse is expected to abide by a code of ethics. The word "ethics" is defined as the conduct appropriate for all members of a group. The American Nurses Association adopted the following version of the Code of Ethics in 1976.

A CODE OF ETHICS FOR NURSES

- To conserve life, alleviate suffering, and to promote health. The nurse does not have the right to make judgments as to the taking of a life. Part of the nurse's responsibility is to be adequately prepared to assist in an emergency or in the usual hospital situation in such a way as to protect the patient against injury or death. Negligence or inability to perform one's duties is as unethical as performing a wrongful act.

- To give nursing care that is not influenced or altered by the personality of the patient, race, social status, religion, or any other external factor. The care given to all patients must be of the same quality, regardless of any personal considerations of the patient or nurse. The nurse must respect the beliefs and customs of the patient.

- To maintain high standards of ethics in personal life and to practice good citizenship.

- To keep up to date with current nursing practice so as to be adequately prepared to give the best possible care to the patient. This includes attending inservice education meetings and maintaining active membership in nursing organizations, as well as reading the current nursing journals and maintaining licensure.

- To keep confidential all information regarding the patient. Although information contained in a patient's chart may be subpoenaed by a court of law, the nurse never voluntarily divulges information of a confidential nature unless the patient's best interests require this to be done.

  In answer to the patient's statement: "I will tell you something if you promise not to tell anyone," the nurse can indicate that the confidence will be kept only if it will not be dangerous to the physical or mental health of the patient. In almost every case, the patient will divulge the information anyway—the patient brought it up because he or she wanted to discuss it. If the nurse promises not to tell anyone and then is given critical information, the nurse is placed in a difficult situation.

- Never to engage in gossip about patients or staff members. (Remember that you may be overheard in the cafeteria or other area. Therefore, it is a wise plan never to discuss patients except in the appropriate area of the nursing station.)

- To do no damage to the public good. This means not using one's position as a nurse or the nursing uniform in any advertising or selling scheme, or as a means of obtaining favors.

- To be a responsible member of society by upholding the laws of that society.

- To make some decisions about nursing care, but never to delegate duties to anyone who is not qualified to perform them. The practical nurse must also remember that he or she is always under the supervision of the RN or physician, and must practice within the bounds of practical nursing. The practical nurse should follow the orders of the physician, yet should question any orders that may seem to be in error.

- To report pertinent information as soon as possible after learning of it, so that the patient will receive the best possible care.

- To know personal limitations and not hesitate to request assistance when necessary. If the nurse does not know how to look up information, it is important to know whom to ask.

- Never to participate in any unethical procedure.

- Never to prescribe treatments or medications or to take harmful drugs.

- To carry out orders with the greatest skill possible. The nurse is expected to abide by the specific rules and regulations of the place of employment. If these rules and regulations are not in accordance with the nurse's code of personal ethics, the question should be discussed with the supervisor. The nurse is also obligated to report unethical practices on the part of a person or institution to the appropriate authorities. It is as unethical to avoid reporting an illegal or unethical practice as it is to participate in this practice. Examples of such conduct include charging a patient for services not rendered, personally using drugs prescribed for a patient, working while under the influence of drugs or while intoxicated, and taking or using supplies assigned to a patient. While the nurse should be loyal to the physician, the patient, and the hospital, it is important to consider the welfare of the patient at all times.

- To serve the employer loyally, give proper notice of resignation, and to give support to the aims of the institution.

- Not to accept tips or gifts from patients. In special situations, the instructor should be consulted for suggestions as to how to handle this situation. It is also improper to borrow anything from a patient.

- Not to burden the patient with your personal problems. The patient needs all his or her available energy to return to wellness.

- In general, not to witness legal papers or wills, particularly while a student.

Suggested References on Nursing

Books

Baly, M. (1986). *Florence Nightingale and the nursing legacy*. Dover, NH: Croom Helm.

Breckinridge, M. (1952). *Wider neighborhoods: A story of the Frontier Nursing Service*. New York: Harper.

Bullough, V., Church, O., and Stein, A. (Eds.) (1988). *American nursing—a biographical dictionary*. New York: Garland.

Carnegie, M. E. (1995). *The path we tread—blacks in nursing worldwide, 1854–1994*. Third Edition. New York: National League for Nursing Press.

Kalisch, P. and Kalisch, B. (1988). *The advance of American nursing*. Boston: Little, Brown.

Kaufman, M. (Ed.) (1988). *Dictionary of American nursing biography*. Westport, CT: Greenwood Press.

Kelly, L. and Joel, L. (1995). *Dimensions of professional nursing*. Seventh Edition. New York: McGraw-Hill.

Kelly, L. and Joel, L. (1996). *The nursing experience: Trends, issues and transitions*. Third Edition. New York: McGraw-Hill.

Pryor, E. (1987). *Clara Barton: Professional angel*. Philadelphia: University of Pennsylvania Press.

Sanger, M. (1938). *An autobiography*. New York: W.W. Norton.

Schorr, T. and Zimmerman, A. (1988). *Making choices, taking chances: Contemporary nursing leaders tell their story*. St. Louis, MO: C.V. Mosby.

151

Siegel, B. (1983). *Lillian Wald of Henry Street*. New York: Macmillan.

Wald, L. (1934). *Windows on Henry Street*. Boston: Little, Brown.

Videos

The following videos are available from the National League for Nursing. They can be purchased or rented. For details, contact the NLN, 350 Hudson Street, New York, NY 10014. Toll free: 1-800/669-9656.

Career Encounters—Nursing. Explores nursing as a career, showing choices from family interaction of home health care to the fast pace of the emergency room. (#42-2380)

Career Encounters—Advanced Practice Nursing. Shows nurses in advanced practice in a variety of settings. Describes preparation for APN roles. (#42-2659)

Nursing in America: History of Social Reform. Renowned nursing historians and educators relate the evolution of American nursing, showing its famous legendary leaders through the years. (#42-2313)

Nursing in America—Through a Feminist Lens. Compares nurses' historic struggle for independence with feminists' battles to empower women. (#42-2435)

Additional Resources for Career Information

Educational Programs and Financial Aid

Annual Guide to Graduate Nursing Education (1995). New York: National League for Nursing Press.

NLN Guide to Undergraduate RN Education (1995). Third Edition. New York: National League for Nursing Press.

Peterson's Guide to Nursing Programs (1994). Princeton, NJ: Peterson's Guide, Inc.

Scholarships and Loans for Nursing Education, 1995–1996 (1995). New York: National League for Nursing Press.

State-Approved Schools of Nursing—RN (1995). New York: National League for Nursing Press.

State-Approved Schools of Nursing LPN/LVN (1995). New York: National League for Nursing Press.

Nursing and Related Organizations

Agency for International Development
US Department of State
Main State Building
2201 C Street NW
Washington, DC 20520

Air Force Nurse Corps
HQ USAF Recruiting Service/RSHN
Randolph Air Force Base, TX 78150

Air National Guard
National Guard Bureau/SG
Room 2E369
The Pentagon
Washington, DC 20310

Air Force Reserve
HQ Air Force Reserve SG
Robbins Air Force Base, GA 31098

Alpha Tau Delta Nursing Fraternity
5207 Mesada Street
Alta Loma, CA 91701

American Academy of Ambulatory Care Nursing
Box 56
East Holly Avenue
Pitman, NJ 08071-0056

American Academy of Nurse Practitioners
Capitol Station, LBJ Building
PO Box 12846
Austin, TX 78711

American Academy of Nursing
600 Maryland Avenue SW
Washington, DC 20024-2571

American Assembly for Men in Nursing
PO Box 31753
Independence, MO 44131

American Association of Colleges of Nursing
One Dupont Circle
Suite 530
Washington, DC 20036

American Association of Critical-Care Nurses
191 Columbia
Aliso Viejo, CA 92656

American Association for the History of Nursing
PO Box 90803
Washington, DC 20090

American Association of Neuroscience Nurses
Suite 204
218 North Jefferson
Chicago, IL 60606

American Association of Nurse Anesthetists
222 South Prospect Avenue
Park Ridge, IL 60068-4001

American Association of Occupational Health Nurses
50 Lenox Pointe
Atlanta, GA 30324

American Association of Office Nurses
109 Kinderkamack Road
Montvale, NJ 07645

American Association of Spinal Cord Injury Nurses
75-20 Astoria Boulevard
Jackson Heights, NY 11370

American Board of Nursing Specialties
c/o American Nurses Credentialing Center
600 Maryland Avenue SW Ste. 100W
Washington, DC 20024-2571

American Cancer Society
1599 Clifton Road NE
Atlanta, GA 30329-4250

American College Health Association
780 Elkridge Road
Linthicum, MD 21090

American College of Nurse-Midwives
818 Connecticut Avenue NW
Suite 900
Washington, DC 20006

American Health Care Association
1201 L Street NW
Washington, DC 20005-4024

American Heart Association
7272 Greenville Avenue
Dallas, TX 75231-5129

American Holistic Nurses' Association
c/o Olson Management Group, Inc.
4101 Lake Boone Trail #201
Raleigh, NC 27607-7506

American Hospital Association
One North Franklin
Chicago, IL 60606

American Indian/Alaskan Native Nurses Association
c/o Erna Burton
Sacaton Service Unit
PO Box 38
Sacaton, AZ 85247

American Journal of Nursing Company
555 West 57th Street
New York, NY 10019-2961

American Medical Association
515 North State Street
Chicago, IL 60610-4320

American Nephrology Nurses Association
Box 56
East Holly Avenue
Pitman, NJ 08071-0056

American Nurses Association
600 Maryland Avenue SW
Suite 100
Washington, DC 20024-2571

American Nurses Credentialing Center
600 Maryland Avenue SW, Suite 100
Washington, DC 20024-2571

American Nurses Foundation
600 Maryland Avenue
Washington, DC 20024-2571

American Occupational Therapy Association
1383 Piccard Drive
Box 1725
Rockville, MD 20849-1725

American Organization of Nurse Executives
840 North Lake Shore Drive
Suite 10E
Chicago, IL 60611

American Physical Therapy Association
1111 North Fairfax Street
Alexandria, VA 22414

American Psychiatric Nurses Association
6900 Grove Road
Thorofare, NJ 08086

American Public Health Association
1015 15th Street NW
Washington, DC 20005

American Radiological Nurses Association
2021 Spring Road
Suite 600
Oak Brook, IL 60521

American Red Cross
430 17th Street NW
Washington, DC 20002-4604

American School Health Association
7263 State Rte 43
PO Box 708
Kent, OH 44240-0708

American Society for Parenteral and Enteral Nutrition
8630 Fenton Street
Suite 412
Silver Spring, MD 20910

American Society of Ophthalmic Registered Nurses
Post Office Box 193030
San Francisco, CA 94119

American Society of Plastic and Reconstructive Surgical Nurses
Box 56
East Holly Avenue
Pitman, NJ 08071

American Society of Post Anesthesia Nurses
11512 Allecingie Parkway
Richmond, VA 23235

Army Nurse Corps Opportunities
Post Office Box 7700
Clifton, NJ 07015-4865

Association of Child and Adolescent Psychiatric Nurses
1211 Locust Street
Philadelphia, PA 19107

Association of Community Health Nursing Educators
5700 Old Orchard
Skokie, IL 60077-1057

Association of Nurses in AIDS Care
704 Stony Hill Road
Suite 106
Yardley, PA 19067

Association of Operating Room Nurses
2170 South Parker Road
Suite 300
Denver, CO 80231

Association of Pediatric Oncology Nurses
11512 Allecingie Parkway
Richmond, VA 23235

Association of Rehabilitation Nurses
5700 Old Orchard Road
First Floor
Skokie, IL 60077

Association of State and Territorial Directors of Nursing
415 2nd Street NE
Washington, DC 20002

Association for Women's Health, Obstetric and Neonatal Nurses
700 14th Street
Suite 600
Washington, DC 20005

Centers for Disease Control and Prevention
1600 Clifton Road NE
Atlanta, GA 30333

Chi Eta Phi Sorority
3029 13th Street NW
Washington, DC 20009

Commission on Graduates of Foreign Nursing Schools
3600 Market Street
Suite 400
Philadelphia, PA 19104-2651

Consolidated Association of Nurses in Substance Abuse
303 West Katella Avenue
Suite 202
Orange, CA 92667

Department of Veterans Affairs Nursing Service
810 Vermont Avenue NW
Washington, DC 20420

Dermatology Nurses Association
Box 56
East Holly Avenue
Pitman, NJ 08071

Division of Nursing
Bureau of Health Professions
5600 Fishers Lane
Parklawn Building, Rm. SC-26
Rockville, MD 20857

Emergency Nurses Association
230 East Ohio
Suite 600
Chicago, IL 60611

Food and Drug Administration
5600 Fishers Lane
Rockville, MD 20857

Frontier Nursing Service
Wendover, KY 41775

Home Healthcare Nurses Association
437 Twin Bay Drive
Pensacola, FL 32534

Hospice Nurses Association
5512 Northumberland Street
Pittsburgh, PA 15217

International Association of Forensic Nurses (IAFN)
6900 Grove Road
Thorofare, NJ 08086

International Council of Nurses
3, Place Jean Marteau
CH-120
Geneva, Switzerland

International Nursing Index
555 West 57th Street
New York, NY 10019

International Society of Psychiatric Consultation Liaison Nurses
437 Twin Bay Drive
Pensacola, FL 32534

Intravenous Nurses' Society
Two Brighton Street
Belmont, MA 02178

Midwest Alliance in Nursing
2511 East 46th Street E3
Indianapolis, IN 46205

National Alliance of Nurse Practitioners
325 Pennsylvania Avenue SE
Washington, DC 20003

National Association for Health Care Recruitment
Box 5769
Akron, OH 44372

National Association for Practical Nurse Education and Service
1400 Spring Street
Suite 310
Silver Spring, MD 20910

National Association of Hispanic Nurses
1501 Sixteenth St. NW
Washington, DC 20036

National Association of Home Care
519 C Street NE
Washington, DC 20002

National Association of Neonatal Nurses
1304 Southpoint Boulevard
Petaluma, CA 94951

National Association of Nurses Practitioners in Reproductive Health
2401 Pennsylvania Avenue NW
Washington, DC 20037

National Association of Orthopaedic Nurses
Box 56
East Holly Avenue
Pitman, NJ 08071-0056

National Association of Pediatric Nurse Associates and Practitioners
1101 Kings Highway North
Suite 206
Cherry Hill, NJ 08034

National Association of Physician Nurses
900 S. Washington Street #g-13
Falls Church, VA 22046

National Association of School Nurses
163 U.S. Route
PO Box 1300
Scarborough, ME 04074

National Association of Social Workers
750 First Street NE #700
Washington, DC 20002-4241

National Black Nurses Association
1511 K Street NW
No. 415
Washington, DC 20005

National Consortium of Chemical Dependency Nurses
1720 Willow Creek Circle
Eugene, OR 97402

National Council of State Boards of Nursing
676 North St. Clair St.
Suite 500
Chicago, IL 60611-2921

National Federation for Specialty Nursing Organizations
Box 56
East Holly Avenue
Pitman, NJ 08071-0056

National Federation of Licensed Practical Nurses
1418 Aversboro Road
Garner, NC 27529

National Flight Nurses Association
6900 Grove Road
Thorofare, NJ 08086

National Gerontological Nursing Association
7250 Parkway Drive
Suite 510
Hanover, MD 21076

National Institute of Nursing Research
National Institutes of Health
9000 Rockville Pike
Bethesda, MD 20892

National League for Nursing
350 Hudson Street
New York, NY 10014

National Nurses Society on Addictions
4101 Lake Boone Trail
Suite 201
Raleigh, NC 27607

National Nursing Staff Development Organization
437 Twin Bay Drive
Pensacola, FL 32534-1350

National Student Nurses' Association
555 West 57th Street
New York, NY 10019-2961

Navy Nurse Corps
Bureau of Medicine and Surgery
23rd and E Street NW
Washington, DC 20037

North American Nursing Diagnosis Association
1211 Locust Street
Philadelphia, PA 19107

Northeastern Organization for Nursing
Department of Nursing
University of New Hampshire
Durham, NH 03824

Nurse Consultants Association
414 Plaza Drive
Westmont, IL 60559

Nurses Christian Fellowship
PO Box 7895
Madison, WI 53707-7895

Nurses Educational Funds
AJN Company
555 West 57th Street
New York, NY 10019-2961

Nurses Environmental Health Watch
181 Marshall Street
Duxbury, MA 02332

Nurses' House
350 Hudson Street
New York, NY 10014

Nursing Organization Liaison Forum
600 Maryland Avenue SW
Washington, DC 20024-2571

Nurses Organization of Veterans Affairs
1341 G Street NW Ste. 1100
Washington, DC 20005

Occupational Safety and Health Administration
200 Constitutional Avenue NW
Washington, DC 20210

Oncology Nursing Society
501 Holiday Drive
Pittsburgh, PA 15220

Peace Corps
P-301
Washington, DC 20526

Project Hope
Project Hope Educational Center
Millwood, VA 22646

Respiratory Nursing Society
5700 Old Orchard Road
First Floor
Skokie, IL 60077

Sigma Theta Tau International
550 West North Street
Indianapolis, IN 46202

Society for Peripheral Vascular Nursing
309 Winter Street
Norwood, MA 02062

Society of Gastroenterology Nurses and Associates
1070 Sibley Tower
Rochester, NY 14604

Society of Otorhinolaryngology and Head/Neck Nurses
439 N Causeway
New Smyrna Beach, FL 32169

Society of Pediatric Nurses
7250 Parkway Drive
Suite 510
Hanover, MD 21076

Southern Collegiate Council on Nursing
592 10th Street NW
Atlanta, GA 30318-5790

The American Association of Nurse Attorneys
720 Light Street
Baltimore, MD 21230

United Nations International Children's Emergency Fund
220 E 42nd Street
New York, NY 10017

U.S. Public Health Service
Department of Health and Human Services
5600 Fishers Lane
Rockville, MD 20857

Visiting Nurse Associations of America
3801 E Florida Street #206
Denver, CO 80210

Western Institute of Nursing
PO Drawer "P"
Boulder, CO 80301-9752

World Health Organization/Pan American Health Organization
525 23rd Street NW
Washington, DC 20037

Wound Ostomy and Continence Nurses Society
2755 Bristol Street
Suite 110
Costa Mesa, CA 92626

State Boards of Nursing

Alabama

Alabama Board of Nursing
RSA Plaza, Suite 250
770 Washington Avenue
Montgomery, Alabama 36130-3900
334/242-4060

Alaska

Alaska Board of Nursing
Department of Commerce and Economic Development
Div. of Occupational Licensing
3601 C Street, Suite 722
Anchorage, Alaska 99503
907/561-2878

Alaska Board of Nursing
P.O. Box 110806
Juneau, Alaska 99811-086
907/465-2544

American Samoa

American Samoa Health Service Regulatory Board
LBJ Tropical Medical Center
Pago Pago, American Samoa 96799
684/633-1222 Ext 206

Arizona

Arizona State Board of Nursing
1651 E. Morten Ave., Suite 150
Phoenix, Arizona 85020
602/255-5092

Arkansas

Arkansas State Board of Nursing
University Tower Building, Suite 800
1123 South University
Little Rock, Arkansas 72204
501/686-2700

California-RN

California Board of Registered Nursing
400 R Street, Suite 4030
Sacramento, California 95814-6200
916/322-3350

California-VN

California Board of Vocational Nurse and Psychiatric Technician
Examiners
2535 Capitol Oaks Drive, Suite 205
Sacramento, California 85833
916/263-7800

Colorado

Colorado Board of Nursing
1560 Broadway, Suite 670
Denver, Colorado 80202
303/894-2430

Connecticut

Connecticut Board of Examiners for Nursing
150 Washington Street
Hartford, Connecticut 06106
203/566-1041

Delaware

Delaware Board of Nursing
Margaret O'Neill Building
P.O. Box 1401
Dover, Delaware 19903
302/739-4522

District of Columbia

District of Columbia Board of Nursing
614 H. Street, N.W.
Washington, District of Columbia 20001
202/727-7468

Florida

Florida Board of Nursing
111 Coastline Drive, East, Suite 516
Jacksonville, Florida 32202
904/359-6331

Georgia-PN

Georgia State Board of Licensed Practical Nurses
166 Pryor Street, S.W.
Atlanta, Georgia 30303
404/656-3921

Georgia-RN

Georgia Board of Nursing
166 Pryor Street, S.W.
Atlanta, Georgia 30303
404/656-3943

Guam

Guam Board of Nurse Examiners
P.O. Box 2816
Agana, Guam 96910
011-671/734-7295(6)

Hawaii

Hawaii Board of Nursing
P.O. Box 3469
Honolulu, Hawaii 96801
808/586-2695

Idaho

Idaho Board of Nursing
P.O. Box 83720
Boise, Idaho 83720-0061
208/334-3110

Illinois

Illinois Dept. of Professional Regulation
320 West Washington Street 3rd Floor
Springfield, Illinois 62786
217/785-9465

Illinois Dept. of Professional Regulation
100 West Randolph Suite 9-300
Chicago, Illinois 60601
312/814-2715

Indiana

Indiana State Board of Nursing
Health Professions Bureau
402 West Washington Street
Room #041
Indianapolis, Indiana 46204
317/232-2960

Iowa

Iowa Board of Nursing
State Capitol Complex
1223 East Court Avenue
Des Moines, Iowa 50319
515/281-3255

Kansas

Kansas State Board of Nursing
Landon State Office Building
900 S.W. Jackson, Suite 551-S
Topeka, Kansas 66612-1230
913/296-4929

Kentucky

Kentucky Board of Nursing
312 Wittington Parkway, Suite 300
Louisville, Kentucky 40222-5172
502/329-7000

Louisiana-PN

Louisiana State Board of Practical Nurse Examiners
3421 N. Causeway Boulevard
Suite 203
Metairie, Louisiana 70002
504/838-5791

Louisiana-RN

Louisiana State Board of Nursing
912 Pere Marquette Building
150 Baronne Street
New Orleans, Louisiana 70112
504/568-5464

Maine

Maine State Board of Nursing
State House Station #158
Augusta, Maine 04333-0158
207/624-5275

Maryland

Maryland Board of Nursing
4140 Patterson Avenue
Baltimore, Maryland 21215-2299
410/764-5124

Massachusetts

Massachusetts Board of Registration in Nursing
Leverett Saltonstall Building
100 Cambridge Street, Room 1519
Boston, Massachusetts 02202
617/727-9962

Michigan

Bureau of Occupational and Professional Regulation
Michigan Department of Commerce
Ottawa Towers North
611 West Ottawa
Lansing, Michigan 48933
517/373-1600

Minnesota

Minnesota Board of Nursing
2700 University Avenue, West #108
St. Paul, Minnesota 55114
612/642-0567

Mississippi

Mississippi Board of Nursing
239 N. Lamar Street, Suite 401
Jackson, Mississippi 39201
601/359-6170

Missouri

Missouri State Board of Nursing
P.O. Box 656
Jefferson City, Missouri 65102
Street Address
3605 Missouri Blvd.
Jefferson City, Missouri 65109
314/751-0681

172

Montana

Montana State Board of Nursing
111 North Jackson
P.O. Box 200513
Helena, Montana 59620-0513
406/444-2071

Nebraska

Bureau of Examining Boards
Nebraska Department of Health
P.O. Box 95007
Lincoln, Nebraska 68509
Street Address
301 Centennial Mall South
Lincoln, Nebraska 68508
402/471-2115

Nevada

Nevada State Board of Nursing
4335 S. Industrial Road, Suite 430
Las Vegas, Nevada 89103
702/739-1575

Nevada State Board of Nursing (2nd Office)
1755 East Plumb Lane, Suite 260
Reno, Nevada 89502
702/786-2778

New Hampshire

New Hampshire Board of Nursing
Health & Welfare Building
6 Hazen Drive
Concord, New Hampshire 03301-6527

New Jersey

New Jersey Board of Nursing
124 Halsey Street, 6th Floor
Newark, New Jersey 07102
201/504-6493

New Mexico

New Mexico Board of Nursing
4206 Louisiana Blvd., NE
Suite A
Albuquerque, New Mexico 87109
505/841-8340

New York

New York State Board of Nursing
State Education Department
Cultural Education Center, Room 3023
Albany, New York 12230
518/474-3843/3845

North Carolina

North Carolina Board of Nursing
3724 National Drive
Raleigh, North Carolina 27612
919/782-3211

North Dakota

North Dakota Board of Nursing
919 South 7th Street, Suite 504
Bismarck, North Dakota 58504-5881
701/328-2974

Northern Mariana Islands

Commonwealth Board of Nurse Examiners
Public Health Center
P.O. Box 1458
Saipan, MP 96950
011-670/234-8950-8954
Telex Number is 783-744,
Answer back code is PNESPN744.

Ohio

Ohio Board of Nursing
77 South High Street, 17th Floor
Columbus, Ohio 43266-0316
614/466-3947

Oklahoma

Oklahoma Board of Nursing
2915 North Classen Blvd., Suite 524
Oklahoma City, Oklahoma 73106
405/525-2076

Oregon

Oregon State Board of Nursing
Suite 465
800 NE Oregon Street, Box 25
Portland, Oregon 97232
503/731-4745

Pennsylvania

Pennsylvania State Board of Nursing
124 Pine Street
Harrisburg, Pennsylvania 17101
717/783-7142

Puerto Rico

Commonwealth of Puerto Rico Board of Nurse Examiners
Call Box 10200
Santurce, Puerto Rico 00908
809/725-8161

Rhode Island

Rhode Island Board of Nurse Registration & Nursing Education
Cannon Health Building
Three Capitol Hill, Room 104
Providence, Rhode Island 02908-5097
401/277-2827

South Carolina

South Carolina State Board of Nursing
220 Executive Center Drive, Suite 220
Columbia, South Carolina 29210
803/731-1648

South Dakota

South Dakota Board of Nursing
3307 South Lincoln Avenue
Sioux Falls, South Dakota 57105-5224
605/367-5940

Tennessee

Tennessee State Board of Nursing
283 Plus Park Blvd.
Nashville, Tennessee 37217-1010
615/367-6232

Texas-RN

Texas Board of Nurse Examiners
9101 Burnet Road
Austin, Texas 78758
512/835-4880

Texas-VN

Texas Board of Vocational Nurse Examiners
9101 Burnet Road, Suite 105
Austin, Texas 78758
512/835-2071

Utah

Utah State Board of Nursing
Division of Occupational & Prof. Licensing
Heber M. Wells Building, 4th Floor
160 East 300 South
Salt Lake City, Utah 84111
801/530-6628

Vermont

Vermont State Board of Nursing
109 State Street
Monpelier, Vermont 05609-1106
802/828-2396

Virgin Islands

Virgin Islands Board of Nurse Licensure
Plot #3 Kongens Gade
St. Thomas, U.S. Virgin Islands 00803
809/776-7397

Virginia

Virginia Board of Nursing
6606 West Broad Street, 4th Floor
Richmond, Virginia 23230-1717
804/662-9909

Washington

Washington State Nursing Care Quality Assurance Commission
Department of Health
P.O. Box 47864
Olympia, Washington 98504-7864
360/753-2686

West Virginia-RN

West Virginia Board of Examiners for Registered Professional Nurses
101 Dee Drive
Charleston, West Virginia 25311-1620
304/558-3596

West Virginia-PN

West Virginia State Board of Examiners for Practical Nurses
101 Dee Drive
Charleston, West Virginia 25311-1688
304/558-3572

Wisconsin

Wisconsin Department of Regulation & Licensing
1400 East Washington Avenue
P.O. Box 8935
Madison, Wisconsin 53708-8935
608/266-0257

Wyoming

Wyoming State Board of Nursing
Barrett Building, 2nd Floor
2301 Central Avenue
Cheyenne, Wyoming 82002
307/777-7601

Glossary

Accreditation   The process by which a voluntary, nongovernmental agency or organization appraises and grants accredited status to institutions and/or programs or services which meet predetermined criteria. The National League for Nursing is recognized by the U.S. Department of Education as the accrediting body for nursing.

Advanced practice nursing   Nursing preparation at the master's degree or higher level. Generally refers to clinical nurse specialists, nurse practitioners, certified nurse-midwives, and certified nurse anesthetists.

Articulated nursing program   The process through which established criteria enable a nurse with one educational credential to advance to a higher academic level. An example would be a nurse with an associate degree advancing to a BSN program.

CAI   Computer assisted instruction. CAI software aims to help user learn concepts or specific content.

Case management   A nursing delivery pattern in which critical pathways or case management plans are used within certain designated timeframes throughout the course of a patient's hospital stay and into post discharge care.

CAT   Computer adaptive testing. A method recently implemented in the NCLEX examination for nursing licensure by the National Council of State Boards of Nursing.

Catheter   A hollow tube inserted into a body orifice to remove or add fluids. It is also used to establish the patency of a body structure.

Certification   A process by which a nongovernmental agency or association certifies that an individual licensed to practice a profession has met certain predetermined standards specified by that profession for specialty practice. Its purpose is to assure various publics that an individual has

179

mastered a body of knowledge, and acquired skills in a particular specialty.

Client   A designation for health recipients in which the focus is on the individual's responsibility for his or her own health habits. Many nurses prefer the term *client* to that of *patient*.

Clinical ladder   A system of recognition and reward to a nurse meeting special criteria at different levels of practice. Also describes the progress of the nurse advancing from one level or step to another.

Clinical nurse specialist   A registered nurse prepared at the master's level or higher in a clinical nursing specialty.

CNM   Certified nurse-midwife. A registered nurse who has met certification standards to practice as a nurse-midwife and whose practice includes prenatal care, labor and delivery management, postpartum care, well women gynecology, and normal newborn care.

CPR   Cardiopulmonary resuscitation. A sequence of steps designed to reestablish normal respiration and circulation after a patient's heart stops beating. CPR involves closed-chest heart massage and aims to establish a clear, open airway.

Credentialing   A method for programs or individuals designed to provide quality assurance to the publics they serve. The most generally recognized mechanisms are accreditation, certification, and licensure.

Defibrillation   The application of an electric current to the heart to treat irregular heart rhythms.

Discharge planning   The extent to which nurses assess the continuing needs of patients early in their hospital stay and before the patient's discharge. They then provide post discharge instructions.

Entry-level program   The basic prelicensure nursing education program for entry into the profession.

Epidemiology   The study of the occurrence, causes, and control of disease in a population.

Geriatric nursing   Nursing care of the aged.

Gerontological nursing   Nursing care of the aged with emphasis on health rather than on disease.

HMO   Health maintenance organization. A system that seeks to control costs by monitoring the delivery of care by limiting access to specialties and costly procedures.

Holistic care   Care of the "whole" person which stresses wellness rather than describing health in relation to diseases.

180

Immunization   An injection or inoculation given to an individual to prevent a specific disease.

Intake-output   A measurement of the amount of fluid and other substances entering the body by ingestion or parenterally. Also indicates the measurement of fluids leaving the body.

IV   Intravenous means within the vein. An intravenous infusion administers fluids into the veins. When blood is given, the infusion is called a transfusion.

Licensure   A process by which an agency of state government grants permission to individuals accountable for the practice of a profession, to engage in the practice of that profession, and prohibits all others from legally doing so. Its purpose is to protect the public by ensuring a minimum level of professional competence.

Managed care   A system that seeks to control costs by monitoring the delivery of care, and by limiting access to specialists and costly procedures.

Medical protocol   An established outline or procedure for implementing a medical treatment.

NCLEX   National Council Licensure Examination. The examination administered to graduates of state approved schools of nursing.

N-G Tube   Nasogastric tube. A catheter inserted through the nose into the stomach, used primarily for liquid nourishment or tube feedings.

Nurse executive   A nurse in a top management position. May also refer to nurses in middle management positions.

Nurse manager   A nurse heading a patient care unit, responsible and accountable for the 24-hour management of that unit.

Nurse practitioner   A registered nurse prepared at the master's degree level or higher, who provides primary health care.

Nursing care plan   An individualized, written plan of care that identifies the specific interventions of the nursing staff to reduce or eliminate patient problems, or to prevent them from occurring.

Nursing diagnosis   Data collected and interpreted by the nurse, which indicates those patient's needs that can be affected by nursing care.

Nursing model   A method of delivery developed and implemented by the professional nurse which focuses on nursing care rather than medical care.

Nursing orders   Written orders for the nurse to follow in meeting the patient's goals.

Nursing Practice Act   Each state's legal definition of the professional practice of a nurse.

Nursing process   A problem-solving approach to nursing problems through assessment, planning, implementation, and evaluation.

OPD   Outpatient department. A component of a health care facility that provides ambulatory care.

Patient education   Provision of appropriate information to patients and members of their social support network.

Physician   A person authorized by law to practice medicine. MD is the abbreviation for doctor of medicine.

Physician's assistant   A person prepared in a formal educational program who works dependently under the supervision of a physician. Referred to as a PA, the provider gives a broad range of health services normally considered the domain of the MD.

Preceptorship   An arrangement in which a student or new staff nurse is assigned on a one-to-one basis to a clinical nurse expert in a health care facility.

Primary health care   Care an individual receives at the first point of contact with the health care system, which may occur in the community, the home, or health care facility. The emphasis is on a long-term relationship among the patient, family, and practitioner.

Primary nursing   Care provided in a health care facility, in which the nurse is responsible as well as accountable for the overall plan of care of an assigned patient, from admission throughout hospitalization over a 24-hour period. The *primary nurse* is the health care provider.

Standing orders   Orders written by the physician for the routine care of the patient.

State Board of Nursing   The state government agency that exercises legal control over the opening and closing of schools of nursing, as well as the licensure of individual nurses.

Third party payer   A source, other than the patient, which fully or partially reimburses the health care costs.

Vital signs   Determinants of the patient's vital processes that include the recording of temperature, pulse, respiration, and blood pressure.

Index

Index

Index

Other Books of Interest from NLN Press

Book Title	Pub. No.	Price	NLN Member Price
☐ **In Women's Experience, Volume II** *Edited by Patricia Munhall*	14-2687	$37.95	$34.35
☐ **African American Voices** *Edited by Ruth Johnson*	14-2631	32.95	29.95
☐ **Peace and Power: Building Communities for the Future, 4th edition** *Peggy Chinn*	14-2697	16.95	14.95
☐ **Annual Review of Women's Health, Volume I** *Edited by Beverly McElmurry & Randy Spreen Parker*	19-2546	37.95	34.35
☐ **Annual Review of Women's Health, Volume II** *Edited by Beverly McElmurry & Randy Spreen Parker*	19-2669	37.95	34.35
☐ **The Path We Tread, Blacks in Nursing Worldwide, 1854–1994, 3rd Edition** *M. Elizabeth Carnegie*	14-2678	30.95	27.95